LIVE LONG, LIVE WELL

SKO '2022

To your continued
personal & professional
Success!

Dwayne

live long, live well

7 Steps to Feel & Look Your Best (No Matter Your Age)

Dr. Laurie Blanscet

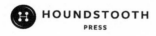

HOUNDSTOOTH
PRESS

LIVE LONG, LIVE WELL

7 Steps to Feel & Look Your Best (No Matter Your Age)

ISBN   978-1-5445-2225-8 *Hardcover*

978-1-5445-2224-1 *Paperback*

978-1-5445-2223-4 *Ebook*

978-1-5445-2226-5 *Audiobook*

I dedicate this book to several wonderful people in my life. I am grateful every day for each one of you.

First, I would like to say thank you to my incredible husband, John, who has been by my side every step of the way. Without him this book would not have been possible. His love, support, and encouragement are beyond words.

I am eternally grateful to my parents for bringing me into this world and for raising me to think for myself, to live with integrity, and to have resilience. Without you, I would not be the person I am today.

I appreciate each one of the phenomenal staff and wellness partners that work alongside me, helping my patients and myself achieve an optimal state of wellness. I love the positive energy that we create together.

I also dedicate this book to every person who has given me the wonderful opportunity of helping them achieve optimal wellness. Seeing you achieve optimal wellness made me realize I needed to share this information so that more people could do the same.

Contents

Disclaimer and Legal Notices

The information provided in this book is designed to provide helpful information on the subjects discussed. This book is not meant to be used, nor should it be used, to diagnose or treat any medical condition. For diagnosis or treatment of any medical problem, consult your own physician. The publisher and author are not responsible for any specific health or allergy needs that may require medical supervision and are not liable for any liabilities, damages, or negative consequences, real or perceived, from the use of this information including any treatment, action, application, or preparation, to any person reading or following the information in this book. References are provided for informational purposes only and do not constitute endorsement of any websites or other sources. Readers should be aware that the websites listed in this book may change.

Preface

While there have been many books written on different aspects of hormone balancing and health in general, I have found that most books are overwhelming to the majority of people. The big picture gets lost in the details that the books review. People are desperate for help, for guidance on optimizing their health, but get frustrated and lost in all the information that is available.

As you will read in the following pages, I am not only a licensed medical doctor, but I have been the patient and have figured out what it takes to achieve optimal wellness on a personal level. I have taken the past fifteen years researching and fine-tuning how to simplify the achievement of optimal wellness.

This book gives you the overview of what it takes to achieve optimal wellness and gives you simple steps that you can easily take. This big-picture view makes it easy for you to do what it takes to feel and look great, for as long as possible.

My goal for writing this book was to assist people from all walks of life achieve optimal wellness: from the person who feels completely out of balance to the person who is in good shape but knows there is a more optimal state of wellness.

Enjoy your journey to an optimal you!!

Introduction

There I was, just a few years into my private practice. I was working the typical long hours of a doctor, rushing through each day with little thought for myself, when I found out I had multiple fibroids (benign tumors) in my uterus. Soon, the pain and irregular bleeding affected everything I did. Rather than listen to my body, I decided a hysterectomy would solve the issue. After all, that was what traditional medicine had taught me. *Diagnose the problem, then fix the problem without delving into the cause of the problem.*

At that point, I was still in a "rush" mindset. Everything was rushed. I needed to rush to get a hysterectomy. I needed to rush to be back to work in two weeks. All I could think of was fixing the issue as quickly as possible. I thought the fast way was the best way.

Boy, was I wrong.

During the surgery, the doctors discovered I had lived through a ruptured appendix. By some miracle, my body had healed itself from the appendicitis and walled off the area to protect my body from the infection. This miracle saved my life but also left behind a diseased, scarred area in my abdomen. Clearly, I had somehow learned to live with extreme inflammation and discomfort, and even thought of it as "normal."

It took me many more years to recognize a simple truth: constant discomfort is not normal.

During the hysterectomy, the doctors attempted to fix the old, diseased area of my intestines and accidentally nicked (cut a small hole in) my bowels. From that point forward, my medical journey began. I was in the hospital three different times, for a total of forty days, and could not work for almost five months. I ended up losing almost thirty pounds and became severely anemic, with a hemoglobin of about eight (should be above twelve). My muscles atrophied as my body "ate" my own muscle to stay alive. At one point, I had pneumonia. At another, I had an allergic reaction to an anesthetic that nearly killed me. The list goes on: an abscess in my abdomen, a blood clot in my left arm, an IV feeding tube for over three months.

I was weak, frail, fatigued, and closer to death than I care to admit.

On the outside, before this happened, I was a seemingly healthy thirty-eight-year-old woman, and yet I almost didn't come out alive. The entire experience was humbling, to say the least.

As horrible as the experience was, I am eternally thankful for having had it. That may sound strange to say, but getting close to death finally woke me up.

MY JOURNEY IN THE HEALTH CARE WORLD

Today, I am an integrative medicine physician with a thriving practice in Murrieta, California. As an integrative physician, I evaluate the whole person and focus on prevention and getting to the root cause of the medical issues a patient is having. Integrative medicine is a proactive arm of medical care. I did not always practice this type of medicine.

In fact, I was not trained at all for this type of medicine in medical school. Instead, I spent hours upon hours learning how to diagnose diseases and how to administer pharmaceutical medications. There was minimal, if any, training on getting to the cause of diseases and preventing illness by utilizing nutrition, exercise, hormone balancing, supplements, toxin avoidance, detoxification, restful sleep, and the mind-body connection.

I graduated medical school in 1996 and finished my family

medicine residency in 1999, becoming board-certified in family medicine. I knew I didn't want to work for someone else, so I took the appropriate steps to open a private family medicine office. I moved from Orange County, California, to Murrieta, California, and started a practice in an area that was growing in population and was more affordable for starting a medical practice.

I always had good intentions. I genuinely wanted to help patients achieve better health, and my practice quickly grew. I hired a physician assistant to help with the workload and saw all types of patients—from children to adults to geriatrics. My patients came to me for everything from a routine physical to a bacterial or viral infection to diabetes and even cancer. I enjoyed getting to know each patient on a personal level.

Over time, it became clear that the way I was trained to practice medicine wouldn't be enough for my patients. I began to question the validity of the medical system more seriously. Should I do what other doctors were advocating? Should I prescribe cholesterol medication without also recommending lifestyle changes? Sure, medication can sometimes help, but it is rarely the long-term answer. Moreover, these medications came with serious side effects.

Putting band-aids on issues by prescribing medication could only go so far. I wanted to be proactive and help my patients prevent problems in the first place, so I spent time counseling each one on preventive care and even helping some get off medications.

I quickly found that insurances do not value this kind of time spent with patients. In fact, health insurance companies only pay based on the number and severity of diagnoses a patient has. They do not pay based on time or diseases prevented. I like to call it "disease" insurance because it is a disease-based system, not a true health-based system. I have also heard it called "sick" insurance because it pays for people to go to the doctor when they are sick, not to prevent sickness.

As I tried to work within this system, I found that truly making a bigger difference in my patients' lives came at a cost. It added hours to my day, and I needed to see more patients to cover my overhead. It also meant I didn't have time to pay attention to my health. I grabbed food that was convenient and fast. I canceled 95 percent of the vacations I planned because I simply could not get away from the practice. Over 50 percent of the time I spent out of the office was taken up by administrative or patient care duties. There was no quiet time to rest and relax.

I was on the merry-go-round of life and forgot that I wouldn't be able to care for others if I didn't care for myself. I lived with daily inflammation that had become so commonplace to me that I could ignore it, just like most people do. I was headed toward a personal medical catastrophe but "felt fine," or that was what I would tell myself. I was "healthy," or so I thought. I was like the majority of people in the world, thinking I was fine when I really was not.

As a result of the months and years of not following a regular self-care program, I ended up on the horrible medical journey I described. I was only seven years into my medical practice, and I almost died.

This couldn't be the best way.

A NEW WAY TO AN OPTIMAL YOU

My experience as a doctor and a patient gave me the spirit to fight the brainwashing found in traditional medicine. I realized I would need to stand up for what is right, not what is commonly taught. So, I began seeking out wellness-minded doctors and organizations that I could learn from and collaborate with. I wanted to completely change my medical practice to one that truly helped people from the inside out, to a practice that I would love and feel proud of. At the same time, I wanted to be truly healthy myself.

The journey did not happen overnight. It took over a year to simply regain my basic "health," which was not optimal health. It took me several more years to obtain optimal health, and I am still learning and improving my approach to health every day.

During this journey to optimal health, I realized that the medical system, as it exists today, is toxic for both patients and doctors. The system either "kills" the patient by "forcing" the doctor to offer substandard care, or it "kills" the doctor by having the doctor spend hours providing the quality of care that is necessary but not rewarded by the insurance system. After my experience, I wondered: *how many caring doctors have been pushed to the "brink of death" to provide proper care for their patients?* As long as medical education is focused on pharmaceutical drugs, and insurance payments are based on diagnosis codes and value reactive medical treatment, the medical field at large will remain a no-win system.

This system should not be designed to simply put out "fires" and control diseases. It should be designed to determine the root cause of the problem and fix it if possible. The doctor and the patient should be allowed to collaborate and work as a team, along with other wellness providers that are needed for that patient to achieve optimal health. Physicians need to be fully invested in the health of their patients, and patients need to understand that true answers may take time and will require taking real, proactive action. We must move beyond the "quick fix" paradigm.

Though I knew I could not change a whole system, I *could*

change my medical practice. I took the time to become properly educated on integrative medicine and treating patients for optimal health. I was ecstatic to find that I was not alone; there was a growing number of physicians who were fighting for the patient and providing quality medical care outside of the insurance system. I was obsessed with getting the information I needed to transform my own health and my health care practice.

In 2012, thirteen years after I started my original practice, I transitioned into an integrative medical practice that I call *An Optimal You*. I believe all of us can achieve optimal health. My practice incorporates concierge medicine, private pay bio-identical hormone balancing, wellness IVs, detoxification protocols, and more. I have also aligned myself with a group of wellness practitioners that offer added support to my patients. I work closely with a life coach, intuitive consultant, hypnotherapist, aromatherapist, personal trainer, and other highly effective wellness practitioners. My own self-care routine includes a healthy diet, regular exercise, bio-identical hormone replacement, quality supplements, daily gratitude journaling, meditation, breathing exercises, going to a float tank every two weeks, taking regular time off work, and using a variety of local wellness services.

I can now provide the appropriate medical care that my patients need without worrying what insurances say I can do, and I can do that without killing myself. In fact, I can do that while maintaining optimal health. I love how I feel and look. I love being in my fifties and feeling better than I ever did when I was in my twenties and thirties. When I come across someone who hasn't seen me for some time, they tell me I have reverse aged. I'm proud to be this kind of example for my patients as I guide them on their path to a wellness mindset and optimal health.

THE CIRCLE OF WELLNESS

On my journey, I've found several components that are critical to achieve and maintain optimal health. I will go over each of these in the chapters of this book.

All the components make up what I call the circle of wellness: *mindset, nutrition, hormone balancing, exercise, supplementation, sleep,* and *toxin avoidance (along with detoxification)*. Everything is interconnected in the circle of wellness. If one piece of the circle is out of balance, it can affect all the other pieces. It is important to address all the components. You might find that you are doing well in one area, but not all of them.

My goal in writing this book is to share the importance of each component in the circle of wellness. Along the way, I will outline easy-to-follow tips so you can know how to get started toward becoming an optimal you. If you would like to have more energy, feel more balanced, and increase the joy and vitality in your life, then this book is for you. This book is designed for people who want to truly live and enjoy their lives for as long as possible. No matter what your age is now, it is never too late to change your wellness path.

Most people focus on "not dying," but I believe that focusing on truly living is the key to a happy and vital life. I believe in living well and dying quick (much later in life, of course!). I experienced what it was like to linger in a hospital, and that is not the way anyone should live out their final days. I will guide you on how to live well and to live a long life. You simply need to be ready to take the necessary action.

As you learn about the components, pick at least one of them to work on. Starting is half the battle. So, start somewhere and improve your health in one area, which will then motivate you to move on to others. Over time, you will have worked on all components in the circle of wellness, and you will be equipped to make specific adjustments that work for you.

I have gone through this process myself and seen miraculous changes in my mind and body. Many of my patients have also embraced the process and achieved optimal wellness for themselves. You can do the same. All it takes is a willingness to change and to take one step at a time.

Here is your first step: read this book, learn, educate yourself on what it takes. As you read, you will be challenged to take specific action steps. Grab a journal or notebook to take notes along the way. Before you dive into the first chapter, take a moment to decide to be unstoppable in pursuing optimal health and becoming an optimal you. The best is yet to come!

Journal Time

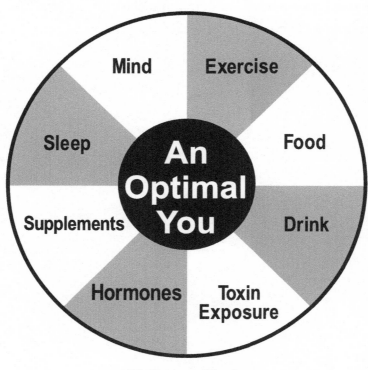

Wellness Circle

CHAPTER 1

The Journey to Optimal Health

"If you do what you've always done, you'll get what you've always gotten."

—TONY ROBBINS, RESULTS/LIFE COACH

"People are asleep. Our job is to wake them up. Most people live, very few are alive."

—MICHAEL BERNOFF, RESULTS/LIFE COACH

All of us entered this world the same way, and we all move through similar developmental stages. In each stage, we learn more about our bodies but don't necessarily change our approach to health. In fact, as teenagers, most of us think we're invincible, that nothing can harm us. We pay little attention to our health and may even do things that harm our health. Even as adults—with a greater ability to choose the life we want for ourselves—few of us wise up and change our habits. Instead, we begin a long journey toward deteriorating health, leading to all kinds of diseases.

Because our brains are wired to avoid discomfort more than they are wired for pleasure, many of us must learn the hard way through a "wake-up call." Even as a trained physician, I was no different.

My wake-up call came in November of 2006. Before this point, I was a board-certified family physician with a thriving private practice. I was happily married and enjoyed my free time. I remember thinking to myself, *How much better could life be?* After all, I was blessed with the ability to make a difference in other people's lives—right?

Unfortunately, the bliss didn't last long. I quickly became busy from morning to night with my work. I was constantly exhausted and was not taking the best care of myself. On the surface I appeared "healthy" but on the inside I was not. I managed to exercise regularly, but my sleep was interrupted, my diet was haphazard, my mind was always going, and my hormones were out of balance.

As I shared in the introduction, I was trying to work in a broken system. I believed in providing quality health care, but doing so came at a cost. I only later recognized that a system that sacrifices the health of the medical provider to provide for the health of the patients is a dysfunctional system. At the time, I was on the merry-go-round—going in circles, trying to keep up, unable to even acknowledge that my regular discomfort was a problem. I was living a reactive life instead of a healthy, proactive life.

Have you ever felt like that?

That you are on the merry-go-round of life, so busy taking care of everything and everyone that you don't have time to take care of yourself? That you are constantly playing catch-up in life? That you are reacting to life instead of proactively planning the life that you desire?

That's exactly where I found myself.

At one point, I remember having intense excruciating pain in my right lower abdomen (below the belly button). I thought to myself, *Maybe I have appendicitis.* But then I "reasoned" myself out of what I instinctively knew. *No, I'm fine.*

The pain eventually subsided, but unbeknownst to me I had a ruptured appendix. This time, my body had miraculously healed itself, but eventually things would catch up with me. I continued to work on the merry-go-round of life, doing what I needed to do without paying adequate attention to my well-being.

Fast-forward about a year. I started having abnormally painful periods. I knew this wasn't normal, and I sought out a gynecologist I trusted. Soon I discovered I had fibroids—benign tumors in the uterus. They were not cancerous, but I also knew I had to do something about them before I "bled to death." At the time, I was not aware of alternative treatments, so I scheduled a hysterectomy. I told my staff I would be out for two weeks and would recover quickly. After all, I was healthy, right?

During the surgery, the doctors found that the ruptured, walled-off appendix had scarred itself in my abdomen. They had to fix it, or it could potentially cause me problems later in life. Since they had not consulted me about that part of the surgery, they woke me up partly through surgery, got my consent, and proceeded to fix the walled-off, diseased area in my abdomen.

Things should have gone well, but they didn't. The surgeon, being human, accidentally nicked my bowel (a part of my large intestine that was near the diseased scarred area). They told me what happened when I woke up, but everything seemed fine, and I was told I could go home from the hospital three days after the surgery.

Right before I was to be discharged home, I ended up so nauseated I couldn't keep anything down. I had a nasal gastric tube (tube from the nose into the stomach that drains stomach fluid) put in and ended up in the hospital for twenty more days. Little did I know that this was only the start of a terrible downhill ride for my health. Because I was one of a quarter million people allergic to the anesthetic used to put the tube in, I lost consciousness and my blood oxygenation dropped dramatically.

Thankfully, the physicians were able to diagnose and treat the issue with an IV infusion of methylene blue. When I regained consciousness, I looked down and saw what appeared to be blue blood being infused into me. Being a *Star Trek* fan, I attempted to make the Vulcan sign. I wasn't very good at it, and I was still groggy. My husband thought I had brain damage when he saw my sad attempt at making the Vulcan sign, but I was simply trying to make a joke. My motto is: *you either laugh or cry, and it's much more fun to laugh at a situation no matter how dire it is*. That motto ended up getting me through the next few months.

During those twenty days in the hospital, I had infected fluid that had to be drained from my abdomen, a blood clot, and pneumonia. I was overjoyed to finally leave the hospital, but my journey did not stop there. After about a week, on New Year's Day, I was watching the Rose Parade and felt excruciating pain in my lower abdomen. After my husband saw me curled up in a ball, he asked me to seek help. Of course, doctors don't always make the best patients. I refused. Thankfully, by some miracle, my gynecologist/surgeon decided to call and check on me. She heard the pain in my voice. I told her I would be fine; she did not believe me. She reiterated that I needed to go to the hospital. I again resisted, but eventually I accepted that I could not *will* myself to be well.

I went to the emergency room, and within a half hour the doctors discovered that I had developed a fistula. My intestinal tract had developed its own little tract to the outside of my abdomen, to the skin, which released pressure. Another obstacle to overcome. I was in the hospital for a week and ended up being discharged home with a colostomy bag that was attached to the newly formed fistula, allowing the rest of my bowels to rest. I also had the joy of being fed by a PICC line (long-term peripheral IV access) since I could not eat. The line was placed in my upper arm and allowed my body to get necessary nutrition via IV.

I would love to tell you my journey stopped there, but no, there was more for me to undergo to fully get a wake-up call. Despite everything I had been through, I was still in a rush to return to work and get back onto the merry-go-round. *After all*, I thought, *I can still see patients with an IV in me.*

Now, looking back, I realize how warped my thinking was. I was completely reactive and not putting myself first. It took me a long time to take full ownership of the fact that not putting myself first actually hurt those around me. Luckily, I did eventually "wake up" and learn.

Have you ever put your health at the back of the line? Putting everyone first except yourself? On the surface it may seem like the right thing to do, but is it? Hopefully, my story shows you that doing this ends up hurting you and the people that you care about.

Before I could get back to work, I had a consultation with a gastrointestinal colorectal surgeon, and she told me that I would need more surgery to fix the problem. I remember her saying I was a "ticking time bomb" and that the problem had to be fixed. Being the great patient I was, I told her that she was wrong, that I would heal, and that I was starting to feel better.

Maybe you can relate to the experience of telling yourself you are fine, when deep down you know you are not. Of course, lying to yourself can't last forever.

Two days after I met with the surgeon, I had so much pain that I had to give her a call. She told me to go to the emergency room and meet her there. Luckily for me, she knew how to fix me. She set me up for surgery and found that my bowels had wrapped around themselves. Had I not had surgery, my bowels would have ruptured and that would have probably killed me. At that point, I was down to 102 pounds at five-foot-four and my hemoglobin was eight (I was dangerously anemic). I was weak and tired and without the physical defenses I had going into the original surgery. I like to joke that I have nine lives like a cat and that this entire medical episode took about four or five of them, but I still have several left...

Thanks to that doctor coming into my life when she did, I was able to recover. She had to remove my right colon, a foot of my small intestine, my gallbladder (the tube feeding had caused a huge gallstone), and my one remaining ovary. This procedure unfortunately thrust me into menopause, but it also saved my life.

After that final surgery, it took me about six weeks to get off the intravenous tube feeding and to be able to eat on my own. I was finally able to go back to work after being off for about five months. It took me another year to regain my health and another few years to achieve optimal wellness—which would ensure that nothing like this would ever happen again to me.

KEY FOR OPTIMAL WELLNESS: TAKE OWNERSHIP OF WHERE YOU ARE AND WHERE YOU WANT TO GO.

Prior to this medical journey, I equated wellness with getting exercise and being a good weight. After this journey, I realized optimal wellness entails much more. To achieve optimal wellness, I needed to address my mindset, sleep, nutrition, hormone balancing, proper supplementation, exercise, and toxin exposures. I could no longer take a haphazard and reactive approach to my health. I had learned the hard way that having optimal wellness is not predetermined; it is a choice.

Throughout this book, I will share what I learned through my journey to not only regain my health but to achieve optimal wellness. I am on a mission to help my patients and now you. Why go through a horrible medical journey that is *preventable*? You don't need to keep reactively responding to sickness. You have a choice.

Achieving optimal wellness doesn't take perfection. It takes a desire to improve and a decision to take steps toward being healthier. To have this desire and make this decision, you must first recognize that *you are ultimately responsible for your health*.

After my journey, people asked me if I would sue the doctor that nicked my bowel. I always said no. That doctor was a human being who was trying to save my life and did everything he could. He didn't cause the problem. The problem was mine. I ignored the ruptured appendix. I decided not to take care of myself and be proactive with my health. I had to take ownership.

And so do you.

What's great about taking ownership for everything is that it gives you back your control. When you are in a victim or blaming mindset, you lose power. If you take responsibility—controlling your choices and future outcomes—you regain your power. Taking responsibility is empowering instead of disempowering.

Note: for the writing activity below and future activities I outline in this book, I recommend using a journal or section of a journal.

What if you started taking ownership for your decisions and choices instead of feeling like a victim? What if you took back the power? What if you recognized that you are in complete control of what you think and do at all moments of your life? This is such an empowering place to be! And you cannot achieve optimal wellness and vitality unless you empower yourself.

Take a moment to think about ways you have let go of your power by blaming others.

Journal Time

No matter what is in your past, no matter what has happened "to you," whatever still holds a negative emotional weight in your life—write it down now. Take as much time as you need to get it all out. Some of these things may be significant traumas. The point of writing them out is not to make them "right," but to release the grip of victimhood, to regain your power.

Next, take a few moments and look at what you have written. No matter how much you felt out of control at that time, recognize that you have a choice to take control over your future now and take a different path.

Take back the power. Decide to own your choices and decisions moving forward.

You can't change the past, but you can change how you think about it. It's much better to come from a place of empowerment than a place of victimhood.

Once you have embraced taking ownership, you are ready to own your future and start the path toward optimal wellness!

WHERE ARE YOU TODAY?

Honesty is key to this first step of taking ownership. It's not about blaming anyone, including yourself. It is about taking stock of exactly where you are. Just like driving a car to a destination, you must first know the place you are starting from to create an appropriate road map to get to the destination.

In your journal, write down where you are today in your

health. Below are a few places to start, but you may write down other factors about your current health particular to you.

- Your weight, your energy level, your vitality
- Your muscle tone and recovery time after exercise
- Your focus, memory, mood, sleep
- What are you doing, or not doing, on a regular basis for your health?
- What are you eating and drinking?
- How much are you exercising?
- How much time do you spend staring at screens (phone, computer, TV)?
- How much time do you set aside to rest and unwind?
- Do you put your health first?

Journal Time

Write down where you are today and be completely honest. There is no right or wrong answer. Put down what comes to mind. This is for your eyes only unless you choose to share it with someone else.

Once you have done that, you can move to the next question.

WHERE DO YOU WANT TO BE?

"It doesn't matter who you are today—it only matters who you are willing to become."

—TOM BILYEU, HOST OF *IMPACT THEORY*

Imagine yourself a year from now. Imagine this has been the best year ever for your health. You have achieved optimal wellness! Write down what you are doing in terms of your health. Write down how you feel, how you look, what you are doing on a regular basis as if it had happened already. Be as detailed as you can about this.

- What are you eating?
- What are you doing for exercise?
- What are you doing for fun and relaxation?
- How is your energy, overall mindset, mood?
- What supplements are you taking consistently?
- How is your sleep?
- Are you putting your health first?
- What is your self-care routine?
- How do you feel on a regular basis?
- How has this positively impacted your relationships? Your work? Your finances? Your life in general?
- What medications have you been able to stop taking?
- How is this improved health giving you a brighter, better future?

Take the time and be descriptive on the health and life that you desire.

If negative thoughts such as "I can't do that" enter your brain, immediately set them aside. This is the time to create the YOU that you desire. You are giving yourself a destination to "drive" toward.

When I was recovering from my medical journey, I focused on feeling vital and energetic, being able to do the things that I enjoyed doing. I had to focus on where I wanted to be if I wanted to recover fully. You must do the same thing to change the trajectory of your health. This exercise will reveal where you can be, and it will motivate you to make the necessary changes. Live into the vision of your future self, and you will create it.

PROGRESS OVER PERFECTION

"Patience and perseverance have a magical effect before which difficulties disappear and obstacles vanish."

—JOHN QUINCY ADAMS

Keep in mind that little things will add up. You may not be able to see your destination clearly quite yet, but once you decide where you want to go, you'll begin naturally taking steps to get there. In my journey, reaching optimal wellness was never about some magic pill. It was about consistently showing up, moving toward my goals one day at a time.

Here's the truth: the miracle for obtaining wellness does not exist outside of you; it lies within you. It comes from the small decisions and choices you make every day. In

2007, I was in the worst health possible. I was sick in every sense of the word. I was thin with hardly any muscle. I had the energy of a slug. I couldn't pick up my cat; she was too heavy at eight pounds. The idea of walking from my bedroom to the living room was too exhausting to think about. Even as I regained my health, I could not even go to the bathroom without assistance. Today, I exercise six days a week and do a combination of yoga, aerobics, and weight training. I have great muscle tone and look great. I sleep wonderfully, and I have great focus and memory. I have an amazing amount of energy, and I love it! I am traveling to fun destinations and scuba diving on a regular basis. I have put my health as a top priority, and as a result I have achieved optimal wellness, which allows me to live the life that I desire! I am enjoying my life and helping my patients enjoy their lives.

It is important to remember that results didn't come overnight.

The little steps, each day, took me from where I was to where I am. I started by simply walking around the house one time. I slowly increased my strength and endurance to where I could walk about a half mile. Eventually, I was able to maintain a consistent exercise regimen. I also worked on my nutrition over time, changing my diet at a pace that worked for me. I added and deleted things over time until I had a meal plan that served me incredibly well. Along the way, I also learned how to balance my hormones with bio-identical hormones. I educated myself about toxins and eliminated toxic products that were around me. I destressed my life and eliminated obligations that did not serve me. I created a day of true rest each week and made sure to set aside regular time to unplug and have fun.

In short, I created the optimal wellness that I have today *over time*. Am I perfect? No. And you don't have to be either. All you must do is consistently move in the right direction.

So, start by being honest about where you are with your health. Then outline where you want to be a year from now. As you read about each component of the circle of wellness, make small action steps daily within each component toward your desired future self. These components are: *mindset, nutrition, hormone balancing, exercise, supplementation, sleep, and toxin avoidance/detoxification*. Focus on progress, not perfection.

As you move forward on this journey to vitality, remember that living is *NOT* the same as not dying. Do not settle for what has become the norm for so many—living in a state of disease or being unwell, also known as not dying. Instead, choose the path to optimal wellness! Choose to live well and live long!

CHAPTER SUMMARY

Own where you are. Make a list of where you currently are with your health. Be complete and honest with this list. Let go of self-judgment; this is about knowing where you are so you can move forward.

Describe the health you want a year from now. Write down everything you are doing to be in that state of optimal wellness and write down how you look and feel. Let go of any doubts and imagine that you had the best year ever in terms of your health.

Progress over perfection matters. Recognize that it is the little actions and choices you make every day that add up to your success. Celebrate the little positive changes you make on a regular basis. Anything you do that moves you in the right direction is the right thing to do.

The wellness circle is the key to living long and living well. It is important to address all the parts within the wellness circle. The components in the wellness circle are: *mindset, nutrition, hormone balancing, exercise, supplements, sleep, and toxin avoidance/detoxification.* The wellness circle lists these topics and helps you remember what areas must be addressed. If you are not feeling well, come back to the circle and see which area needs adjusting.

"Your life is the sum result of all the choices you make, both

consciously and unconsciously. If you can control the process of choosing, you can take control of all aspects of your life. You can find the freedom that comes from being in charge of yourself."

—ROBERT FOSTER BENNETT

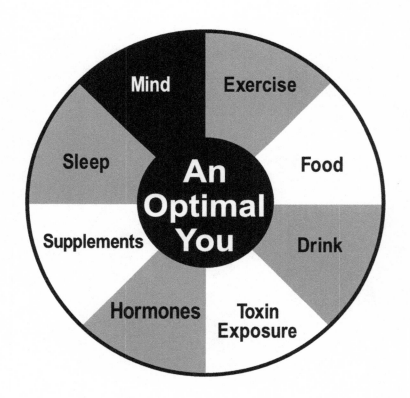

CHAPTER 2

The Power of a Healthy Mindset

"Having a healthy mindset gives you the ability to do whatever you need to do to achieve your goals—your dreams with deadlines."

—JOHN GRANT, LIFE/RESULTS COACH

"Attitude is a little thing that makes a big difference."

—WINSTON CHURCHILL

Have you ever stopped to think about how closely associated your mind and body are? Though we may not take time to recognize this reality, we live by it every day. For example, if you screamed out at me that something was about to attack me, my mind and body would immediately react. I would go into a protection mode and do whatever was needed to save my life.

When threatened, we go into "fight, flight, or freeze" mode. No matter the response, our bodies and minds are working together, without us even noticing.

Of course, it's not every day we are attacked, but our minds and bodies respond in a similar way when we feel stressed or anxious. Think of the last time you felt stressed or anxious. When this happened, your body released hormones that caused your heart rate and breathing to increase, your blood pressure to rise, and your muscles to tense up. This physical reaction was the same fight-or-flight stress response. This physical body reaction came because of your mind perceiving the stress and directing the body to have a response.

There is absolutely no question that the mind affects how the body reacts. Entire books explain the mind-body connection. There's much more to explore on the topic, but for now it is important to simply acknowledge that this connection exists and affects everything we do in life.

Prior to my wake-up medical journey, I was in a stressful state of mind. Of course, I loved helping patients, but I was under a constant state of stress. I worried about everything. I worried about giving my patients the best medical care while covering the expenses of my practice. I worried about how my patients were doing. I worried about personal obligations. And the list goes on.

Being in this state of mental stress created changes in my physical body that were not conducive to optimal wellness. Once I recognized my mindset was a major component of the circle of wellness—a major factor for why I had almost died at the age of thirty-eight—I was able to get to work on fixing that component.

Think of the last time you felt stressed, overwhelmed, or anxious. Did you realize the effect that had over your physical body? Did you ever think about the fact that your headache, stomach pain, muscle pain, high blood pressure, elevated blood sugars, or ultimately a more serious disease could be related to your state of mind? Now is the time to give this some thought.

Again, the point is not to blame yourself; it's to recognize the power of your mind so you can know how to utilize it to help you instead of harm you.

As a physician, I have personally witnessed patients who did not get better until they were given the proper words and encouragement. Their health improved by what seemed like a miracle. On the reverse side, I have seen patients whose anxiety and stress caused them to deteriorate physically. The mind is a powerful tool, and when used correctly, it can assist your body to heal. When used incorrectly, it can make your body ill and keep you ill.

In the late 1800s to early 1900s, there was an apothecary (now known as a pharmacist) named Émile Coué. What was interesting about Coué was that his patients were getting better at a higher rate than the patients of other apothecaries. When asked what he was doing, Coué stated that he asked his patients to repeat out loud to themselves, on a regular basis, the following:

"Every day and in every way, I am becoming better and better!"

By saying this simple, repetitive statement of positivity and healing, his patients really did get better. It seemed like witchcraft, but it was not. Coué was tapping into his patients' minds and using them as tools to instigate physical changes in their bodies. The patients' changed mindset didn't fix everything, but it did make a significant impact on a lot of their lives.

Coué observed that the main obstacle to this statement working was willpower. For the method to work, the patient had to refrain from making an independent judgment, such as telling themselves that the statement wouldn't work. When a patient did that, they let their will (conscious mind) impose its own views on the unconscious mind, and the healing process was stalled. To be successful, the patient had to abandon their conscious thinking and instead put focus on their imagination to allow the mind-body connection to work to its full potential.

Remember writing down where you want your health to be a year from now? By doing so, you are using the power of imagination. You must be able to see yourself in optimal wellness to point your mind and body in the right direction. Of course, you also need to take other action steps to get there, but pointing in the right direction makes the journey easier and achievable.

The mind-body connection can be further illustrated by the placebo effect. The placebo effect is when someone responds favorably to a treatment that can't be attributed to the treatment itself; the positive response must therefore be due to the patient's belief in the treatment. For example, a patient is given a sugar pill that has no physical benefits on blood pressure, but the patient's blood pressure improves. That's the placebo effect at work. For decades, the medical field has discounted the placebo effect. However, science has shown the placebo effect can sometimes be as effective as traditional treatment protocols. Why should we ignore the power that the mind has on the physical body, especially when it comes without the side effects of traditional medicines?

The mind-body connection is such a powerful tool, and you might be wondering how this works.

Here's a brief explanation: When you have a thought (a physical thing), it literally produces a chemical command in the brain. The cells of the body then respond to the chemical command. The cells regain proper functioning simply because they are given the proper command.

During my own medical journey, I saw the power of the mind-body connection and the importance of utilizing the proper mindset. When I first found out about the fibroids in my uterus, I spiraled downhill. My mind was focused on not dying and getting back to all the things that I had to do. I even tried to work from my hospital bed. By the time I had my last surgery, I started to heal.

What changed?

I finally stopped fighting reality, which decreased my stress and allowed me to focus on my health. Prior to the final surgery, I kept having my staff push patients back about two weeks at a time. I was so caught up in what I had to do and the stress of it all that I did not allow my mind (and therefore my body) to focus on healing. Finally, after the final surgery, I switched my mindset. I had my staff cancel my patients for the next eight weeks. I succumbed to the reality that I needed time to heal. Doing that allowed me to stop focusing on rushing back to work and to refocus on healing. It was only then that I truly started to heal from the inside out.

I have heard the same general story as mine from my patients through the years, with only the specific details altered. Most everyone feels that they have no choice. They feel they must stay in the mental state of stress, pressure, and anxiety.

Do you feel pressed into a corner without a choice? Do you believe that you must sacrifice your health to accomplish whatever you must get done?

The truth is you do have a choice.

I found this out the hard way, and I'm sharing my experience so you can choose the right mindset before you face a serious medical issue. Even if you have already faced, or are facing, a serious medical issue, there is still time to choose a healthy mindset.

Once I took the steps to adjust my mindset and no longer lived in a state of stress or fear, no matter what was going on around me, I found my way to healing. Today, I have a thriving medical practice, but I don't let stress and anxiety have the final say. I have found how to be healthy inside and out while still having a productive life, and it started with a healthy mindset.

READY FOR A NEW HEALTHY MINDSET?

Would you like to create a mindset that serves you no matter what is going on in your life?

Now is the time to start. If not now, when?

You now realize that any change in your body starts with changing your mind. Your mind and body are powerful allies. How you think will affect how you feel and how your body functions.

There is power in starting now. Choose today to change your mindset. Make a firm decision to have a healthier mindset. Once you do, you can use the specific steps below to create the positive healthy mindset you need. The best part is that you are in 100 percent control of your mindset.

So, what do you need to do to change your mindset?

BE AWARE OF WHAT YOU FEED YOUR MIND

First, you must realize your mind is wired to look for dangers and keep you alive. Throughout human history, it has been more critical for our survival to recognize dangers and avoid them than to go toward things that were pleasurable. Still today, we are often drawn toward stressful things, like watching news or hearing about negative events.

However, if you surround yourself with negative things like news or toxic people, your body will respond as if a real physical threat was present. Your mind does not understand the difference between a real physical threat, such as a saber-toothed tiger trying to kill you, and a mental threat, such as watching something negative on news. Both the real physical threat and the mental threat create a mental command to your body that it must defend itself. A chemical message is sent to your cells; the fight, flight, or freeze response is initiated. Our bodies were never meant to experience such heightened stress all the time. When we experience mental stressors daily, optimal wellness is not possible.

The good news is that even though our mind is trained to look for the negative, we can train it to look for the positive as well. This does not mean we lose our ability to react to a real physical threat. If something physically threatens you, your mind and body will be fully capable of reacting appropriately. Training your mind to see the positive will simply help your body receive more healing commands so you can achieve optimal wellness. Remember how Émile Coué's daily statement was so effective for his patients? A simple statement, with belief in your mind, can command the body to heal.

If you feed your mind negative, stressful thoughts, they create illness-promoting commands within the body. If you want to live in a state of optimal wellness, you must feed your mind positive thoughts.

How can you do that? Here are some practical steps you can take today.

AVOID WATCHING NEWS.

News is no longer investigational reporting with facts. It has become a dramatic show with a few facts here or there. All news stations know that negativity sells. They play to our mind's desire to look out for dangerous things. Think about it: Have you ever walked away after watching the news and felt good? Do you feel compelled to watch the news, feeling like you must watch to stay informed? Do you ever wonder why you are addicted to watching something that makes you feel bad and doesn't give you useful information?

I encourage you to experiment and avoid watching all news for at least a week. Then assess how you feel. I would bet that you will feel lighter and happier. Why not choose to feel better?

You can still get facts by researching things on your own. And believe me, if aliens land, you will know about it.

By avoiding watching the news, you avoid the excess drama associated with it. Unless you like watching things that negatively impact your mindset, stop watching the news. If you absolutely must watch, limit your watching time to no more than ten minutes a day, and never start or end your day with the news.

AVOID OR MINIMIZE GOING ONTO SOCIAL MEDIA SITES.

If you do go onto social media sites, post positive things about you or your life, positive quotes, things that can impact other people's lives in a good way. Keep the rest for conversations with a trusted friend, counselor, or life coach. It's important to avoid getting engaged in negative debates online. Do not follow or friend anyone who insists on being negative.

If you still want to use social media, limit yourself to no more than ten to twenty minutes of social media per day, avoid getting on a social media site first thing in the morning or later at night, and pick at least one day a week where you avoid social media 100 percent.

PAY ATTENTION TO THE WORDS THAT YOU SAY.

Are you regularly saying "I can't, I won't, I'm not good enough, I'm useless, I hate, it's impossible, that was stupid," or similar phrases? We are all human, and we have all said these words aloud or to ourselves.

Can you see how negative these words are? They give your mind and body the wrong directions.

Why not change what you say to "I choose, I am enough, I'd like to, it's possible, that was one way to do it," or something else that's positive?

Words do matter—not only the words that you say out loud but also those you say inside your mind that nobody else hears. This is what we call self-talk. Pay attention to both.

By changing what you say to more positive words, you will be giving your mind and body more positive instructions. This may seem insignificant. It is not. It is significant because it is the little things that add up over time and they matter.

You may still be thinking this is silly and won't help. Why not look at it in a different way? What is the harm in thinking more positively? How could your life improve by choosing your words more wisely when talking to yourself and others?

Now, think about the potential harm if you continue making negative comments to yourself and others.

Who does it hurt if you continue with negative words? You and those around you.

Who does it help if you change to more positive words? You and those around you.

Would you rather have a negative or positive impact on yourself and others? The choice is yours.

Now is a great time to take out your journal and write down common negative words or phrases that you say or think to yourself. Once you have done that, write down more positive words or phrases that you could say or think in their place.

Journal Time

Pay attention to what you say and think. When you find yourself using a negative word or phrase, stop yourself and change to the more empowering word or phrase. When you pay attention to what you say and think on a regular basis, these new empowering words and phrases will become your new normal and you will find yourself having a healthier mindset.

READ, WATCH, AND LISTEN TO THINGS THAT PROMOTE A POSITIVE STATE OF BEING.

Today, you have so many options. Check out free YouTube videos and podcasts that offer tips on living and thinking better. Explore the wide variety of e-books and printed books on subjects that improve your life. At the end of this book, I will list some of my favorites. Search out sources of positive information and read, watch, or listen to them. You will feel uplifted, which creates a healthy state of mind.

TRAIN YOUR MIND TO BE IN A STATE OF GRATITUDE

When we are living in gratitude, we can't at the same time

be in a state of fear, anxiety, or depression. Gratitude is a positive state of mind and allows our mind to give more healing directions to our body. Besides, being in a state of gratitude simply feels better. Would you rather feel worse or better? Again, the answer seems obvious, but the choice is really yours.

The following are some practical ways to stay in a state of gratitude.

START A GRATITUDE JOURNAL.

Journal Time

This is simple and easy to do daily. Get a separate journal for this. In your gratitude journal, write three things down every morning that you are grateful for. By doing this one simple task, you will be training your mind to look for the great things around you. Of course, there are always things that can hurt us and that are not so positive. But there are also always things that are beautiful and wonderful. No matter what is going on in our lives, this is true.

When I was in the hospital starting to heal, I began to focus on gratitude. I was grateful that I was alive and breathing. I was grateful to have a wonderful, supportive husband who was by my side no matter what. I was grateful for the patients who were still there for me when I returned. Each day, I had at least three things to be grateful for.

Simply waking up each day is something to be grateful for. What you write down each day can be very simple or more complex. You can write down things that you have or things that you wish to have and are grateful for. There is no right or wrong when it comes to gratitude. The important thing is to be consistently writing in your gratitude journal daily.

I personally like using the five-minute gratitude by Intelligent Change (you can easily find this online at www.intelligentchange.com). It starts each day with a wonderful quote or a challenge, and it goes beyond writing down the three things to be grateful for each day by adding in a daily affirmation, among other things.

Would you rather look at the positive part of life or the negative? What do you think serves your mind and body better?

By developing an attitude of gratitude, you will train your mind to find peace and calm no matter what is going on around you. This is a powerful tool, and it will allow you to not only survive but thrive in today's world.

SPEND A FULL DAY APPRECIATING THE THINGS AROUND YOU.

When you shower, appreciate the warm water that you have. Appreciate the feeling of the clothes on your body, the air on your face, the taste and smell of the food as you eat it, and all the other things that you see, feel, and hear throughout the day.

As you go through your day, focus on appreciating and seeing the things around you. We take so much for granted, and it is important to remind our mind that there are beautiful, wonderful things around us all the time. By doing this, you train your mind to look for the good and in turn, train your body to heal instead of existing in a state of illness.

Do this for a full day this week, and then incorporate the practice into every day from this point forward.

UNPLUG REGULARLY AND CREATE A QUIET SPACE FOR YOUR MIND

In today's world, most people are so busy in that merry-go-round of life that they don't take time to enjoy life.

You may currently be where I was in 2006, thinking that everything is okay. But deep down you know that you are not okay. It is easy to put on the façade that everything is okay when it is not. We are expected to work hard and produce. We are not taught how to take proper care of ourselves so that we may live in optimal wellness. I had to learn how to practice self-care, and I know I am not alone.

When was the last time that you enjoyed quiet time? Have

you recently taken the time to simply sit quietly and just breathe?

Everyone needs time to unplug, but if that very thought stresses you out, you desperately need it. I know because I used to be that person. The thought of sitting still and having quiet time felt like torture to me. I thought that if I sat still, I may never get back up. It was the opposite. By not sitting still and resting appropriately, I was leading myself down the path of physical destruction. Now I spend quiet time on a regular basis, not because I feel bad, but because I want to keep feeling amazing! That is the difference between someone just going through life, not dying, and someone who embraces life and truly lives.

I have learned to set aside time on a daily and weekly basis to allow my mind and body to reset. This gives me a sense of calm and peace and allows me to be proactive with the things that are going on around me instead of being reactive. I do not stress about the things that occur around me like other people. That is because I have learned how to build a mental defense by practicing the things that I am teaching you. These tools work. It is up to you to choose to utilize them.

EACH MORNING, TAKE SOME TIME TO JUST BREATHE AND BE PRESENT.

Take at least a minute if that's all you have. Or take ten

minutes, a half hour, or more. Take the time that you have, and sit quietly, breathing in and out slowly. Just be with you and sit quietly. This is best done outside, before you start your day. Breathe in and out, slowly, and deeply, quietly being present with the moment at hand. You will be amazed at how much better your days will be when you start them with a moment or more of quiet breathing.

It is also great to follow this quiet breathing time with a positive affirmation. You can create your own empowering affirmations or simply say aloud, "Every day and in every way, I am becoming better and better!" It is a proven statement that will serve you well.

ON A WEEKLY BASIS, HAVE AT LEAST ONE DAY THAT YOU SET ASIDE TO COMPLETELY UNPLUG.

This is a day to get away from the phone and computer work, get away from obligations, and spend however you wish. This is a day with no plans, no to-do list; it is a day of your choosing. Do anything that regenerates your mind and soul.

At first it may seem difficult to do this, but I promise it gets easier. The world will still be there, and your to-do list will wait for you. Take care of your mind and body, and your mind and body will be in top shape to do the things you wish to get done in life.

TURN OFF YOUR PHONE ON A REGULAR BASIS.

Wait to turn on your phone for at least an hour or two after waking up. It is wonderful to take the first hour or two after awakening to take care of your mind and body. It prepares you for the day.

Be sure to turn off your phone a few hours before you go to sleep. This will enhance your ability to have a quality night's sleep and help your mind destress.

If turning off your phone creates stress in your mind, it is time to face facts that you are probably addicted to your phone. It is critical to be able to unplug from your phone on a regular basis. The buzzes and rings can create a mental stress that is perceived as a physical threat by your mind and body. I personally grew up before cell phones existed and somehow I survived, as did my peers and parents. We can survive without our phones always turned on. I have come to enjoy my one day a week with my phone turned off and having it off in the morning and later evenings. It is wonderful to reconnect with yourself and those that you live with.

On that note, I also advise keeping alerts turned off when your phone is turned on, checking it on your timetable, and not feeling obligated to respond immediately to texts, calls, or emails (unless your job depends on it). The goal here is to decrease the amount of stimulus to your mind. If you must have your phone on for work, be sure to get separate work and personal phones. That way you can avoid business matters interfering with your time off work.

The bottom line is that you must have time away from being overconnected to the world and have more time connected to yourself and the people who live with you.

Take out your journal and write down ways that you can unplug on a daily and weekly basis. Think about how you can fit them into your life and write down your plans to do this. Then put them into your calendar.

Journal Time

FOLLOW THROUGH

Remember to be aware of what you feed your mind, train your mind to be in a state of gratitude, and unplug regularly. I have been following these three key points for a long time now. The transformation these practices can have on the mind and body is absolutely amazing. It may take some time for you to develop these habits to change your mind-set, but it is well worth it. The payoff is huge.

Remember, it is not about perfection; it is the positive daily progress you take that will lead to your success. Make small positive changes utilizing each of the key points I shared in this chapter. Start with one or two of the action items and add to them over time. By making small positive changes on a regular basis, you will find yourself achieving the health that you desire.

All the action items that I have listed cost no more than an investment of time. The best part is that the only side effects are feeling more balanced, calm, and happy. When you feel this way, your body functions more optimally.

Remember, it is always a choice: choosing to do the things that lead us to the path of wellness or choosing to do the things that lead us to the path of illness.

When you choose to adjust your mindset, you will be amazed at how easily your body follows.

If you need additional guidance with adjusting your mindset, I advise enlisting the aid of a life coach. A knowledgeable life coach can be invaluable in assisting you in adjusting the words that you use and in achieving a wellness mindset.

If you find yourself troubled by past traumas or unhelpful beliefs that you cannot shake, I have found that utilizing the services of a clinical hypnotherapist can be a great help. A hypnotherapist can help you get past the conscious mind and tap into the power of the subconscious mind.

If you don't have any of these wellness practitioners in your area, you may access the practitioners that I work with. Most of them can treat clients anywhere in the world. They are listed under the Wellness Partners page at www. anoptimalyou.com.

CHAPTER SUMMARY

Be aware of what you feed your mind. Pay attention to your words and change what you say to yourself and others. Be positive! Avoid watching or listening to the news. Minimize or avoid your exposure to toxic people and social media. Watch, listen to, and read positive things that improve your life.

Have an attitude of gratitude. Each day, write three things you are grateful for in a gratitude journal. Appreciate the things around you. Start each day sitting outside and spend a few minutes having gratitude for your life and body.

Learn to quiet your mind. Unplug on a regular basis. Spend time each morning quietly breathing and being present with the moment. Set aside one day a week with no plans. Avoid turning on your phone immediately after awakening and turn it off a few hours before bed. Meditate whenever you can.

Enlist the help of a life coach if you would like assistance in developing a healthy mindset.

"Nothing is impossible. The word itself says 'I'm possible.'"

—AUDREY HEPBURN

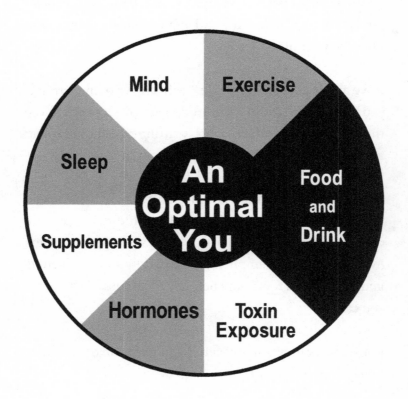

CHAPTER 3

Nutrition

THE PHYSICAL FOUNDATION

"By choosing healthy over skinny, you are choosing self-love over self-judgment."

—STEVE MARABOLI

"The doctor of the future will no longer treat the human frame with drugs, but rather will cure and prevent disease with nutrition."

—THOMAS EDISON

The food that we eat is an important part of the circle of wellness. If you don't eat the right foods, it is impossible to have optimal wellness. The great news is, it is not as hard as you might think it is.

I would love to tell you that I have always eaten well. After all, I'm a physician. I should know the importance of eating well. Sadly, medical education does not put a lot of emphasis on nutrition—at least not when I went to school. I could probably count on two hands how many hours of nutritional education I received. But even if I had the education, would that have changed my habits?

How many of us truly eat in the manner our bodies require? Let's face it, most people eat for pleasure and not for purpose. If you want to have optimal wellness, that must change.

I was aware that nutrition was important, but in my teens, twenties, and even into my thirties I was able to eat pretty much anything I wanted and not notice an apparently negative effect such as being overweight. I could stay within a good weight eating things like Frosted Flakes, tacos, pizza, nachos, pasta, and sweet breads. I was the "appropriate" weight for my height, but that didn't mean I was healthy.

You see, I was a skinny fat person. On the outside I looked thin and in "good" shape; on the inside I had more body fat than muscle mass. That is what I call a skinny fat person: someone who is at a good weight per the scale but has an unhealthy body composition—the fat and muscle ratio. I was doing the healthy things like exercising and drinking only water, but I was not eating well.

What I didn't realize was that my lack of attention to a healthy meal plan was causing inflammation in my body and affecting me in ways I was not aware of. I had gotten used to having stomach pains on a regular basis. I thought it was just the way it was and didn't associate the pain with the foods I ate. I later learned the pain was linked to eating ingredients that were not healthy for me. At one point, I was even told that I probably had Crohn's disease (a chronic inflammatory bowel disease). The illness was not bad enough to need medication, and it was manageable. Or was it?

Because my body was inflamed and my intestines were "upset," I didn't even recognize when my appendix ruptured. Had I been eating properly, not only would I have been feeling better on a regular basis, but I would have caught the appendicitis because I wouldn't have been so familiar with pain.

Consider your daily experience. Have you learned to live with a constant bloated feeling? Have you learned to live with regular headaches, body aches, fatigue, or unexplained rashes? Have you even been diagnosed with an autoimmune disease?

If you have answered yes to any of these, the food you are eating is likely causing inflammation inside your body. In fact, even heart disease, cancers, and other chronic diseases have been linked to inflammation.

Many patients have told me there is no way they could be intolerant to a food they have eaten all their lives. I can tell you from personal experience and from treating many patients over the years that you can react to foods you have eaten all your life. In fact, many of the foods we crave are the very foods that cause inflammatory changes in our bodies.

When we eat food that causes an inflammatory reaction on a daily or regular basis, we don't notice until the offending food is taken away.

We learn to live with things in all kinds of ways. Imagine, for example, that I tapped the side of your arm gently and repeatedly. After a while, you might tune me out.

Now imagine if I suddenly socked you in the arm. You would notice that, wouldn't you?

The first scenario is similar to what happens when you eat foods on a regular basis that are causing inflammation. You adapt to them and allow them to continue to bother you. Your conscious mind essentially ignores them by adapting to the presence of continual inflammation. Your body is inflamed but you are not consciously aware of it. You basically get used to your body not feeling great; it feels "normal" to you. Most people have learned to live with an inflamed body and are not even aware.

The second scenario is similar to what happens when you don't eat those foods, and then after a while you do eat a food that's inflammatory for you. You notice it!

Common inflammatory foods are dairy, wheat, corn (especially high fructose corn syrup), sugar, processed meats, and beef. There are more foods that can be inflammatory, but these are the most common.

KNOW WHEN FOODS ARE HEALING OR TOXIC FOR YOUR BODY

We all have different food tolerances. There is not a specific food that bothers everybody in the same way. The exception to that is sugar. There is no one on earth that sugar is good for. Sugar is inflammatory and should be eliminated, or at least greatly reduced, in your meal plan.

You will need to find the foods that work the best for you. The Whole30 is a great place to start, and the plan is easily accessible online for free. The Whole30 is not a get-thin-quick plan. Instead, it guides you to eliminate the top inflammatory foods, and drinks, for 30 days. This allows your body to reset. The plan is not easy, but it's a quick way to determine the inflammatory foods in your meal plan.

The Whole30 can be a bit overwhelming for some people. You can also take a more gradual approach to eliminating inflammatory foods. Often, you may have your own thought about what foods are bothering you. If you think you have an idea of what foods bother you, take a moment and write them down now. You can also keep a diary of what you eat and the symptoms that you experience to determine foods that bother you.

Once you have a list of foods that may be bothering you, pick one food and eliminate it for three to four weeks and assess how you feel with that food out of your system. Then slowly reintroduce that food and assess how your body and mind feel when it is reintroduced. This is a slower process but can be easier to follow. Journal how you feel along with what you eat to help you pinpoint what foods you should avoid.

Dr. Gundry discovered a list of inflammatory foods that may appear to be healthy on the surface. You can do an internet search and easily print his list of foods that he advises are safe to eat and foods to avoid. If you need help identifying inflammatory foods, this list could help you. Eat from the foods on the yes list and avoid the foods on the no list. I have found his food list to be comprehensive and quite helpful.

There is no miraculous diet out there for everyone. There is not *one* answer for everyone. The key is to be aware that there are inflammatory foods and to pay attention to how your mind and body react to the food you eat. This is a process; it may take time for you to figure everything out.

Early in my recovery process, I started with foods that were easier to eliminate and eventually was able to eliminate wheat and cheese from my diet (two of my previous favorite foods). By doing the elimination process, I found out that rice, wheat, corn, beef, and cheese were not my friends. These foods were causing inflammation in my body. It took me about a year to eliminate them from my diet completely, but once I did, I found that my abdominal pains were gone. After cleaning up the foods that I eat, I no longer live with mental fatigue or stomach bloating. The negative side effects do not return unless I eat one of those foods. I would never miss a ruptured appendix feeling the way I do now!

We are all human, so we sometimes eat things we know we shouldn't. The good news is that when your body reacts to the food, it will remind you not to eat those foods. This reduces your desire for them. When I ate a food that I shouldn't have a few months ago, I was amazed at the effect it had on my body. I felt slightly drunk. I don't ever drink any alcohol, but the food completely altered my mind and body as if I had consumed alcohol.

You may be eating food that is affecting you physically and/ or mentally and not even know it. Once you eliminate it, your body is cleansed of the chronic inflammation and you will notice when you eat it. If that happens, avoid beating yourself up. Embrace the fact that it is a wonderful learning experience! Learn from it and make better choices in the future.

We all have our favorite foods and foods that we don't want to give up. Often when I talk about food with patients, a resistant wall goes up and they refuse to listen. Therefore, we must start with mindset. When you have a healthy mindset, you will be able to accept the changes you need to make and eliminate foods that you currently love. I used to love cheese and breads, but I no longer eat them because they don't serve me.

If you had told me fifteen years ago that I would not be eating any wheat, corn, rice, or cheese, I would have laughed in your face. But here I am, doing exactly that. I had to change my mindset first to realize the critical impact food was having on my health. This is a process, and it takes time. Remember the motto: progress over perfection. Be patient with yourself as you make these changes.

If you are struggling with the thought of never eating food that you love again, it's time to think differently. I felt that way about both bread (wheat products) and cheese, and I was able to eliminate them from my meal plan without any regrets. A little trick that helped me was telling myself that I would stop the food for a set period of time and that it was not forever. If you tell yourself something is forever, it is hard to ever get started on that path.

Another trick is to give yourself small goals to achieve so you can go from one small goal to another. When I told myself that I would not eat the food for a day, I could then go a week without it, and then a month. If I had a craving for that food, I would move my body and change what I was doing. I would tell myself that I could not eat that food for the next five minutes. The craving would subside, and I would move on. Once that month was up, I paid close attention to any difference in how I felt, mentally and physically. Then I reintroduced the food and noted how my mind and body reacted. If I had an obviously negative reaction to a food, I would mentally associate the discomfort with that food. Sometimes I had to repeat eating the food, experiencing the discomfort, and re-associating the discomfort with the food. Eventually the association would stick, and I no longer desired that food.

If you have an addiction to a certain food that you need to try eliminating from your diet, try this trick. It worked for me, and it has worked for many of my patients.

As you clean up your meal plan and avoid the foods that your body does not tolerate, you may find that you can eat some foods that you previously thought bothered you. As your body becomes less inflamed, the foods that may have once irritated your body—because of your overall inflammatory status—will no longer bother you.

As a final note here, you can take a food allergy test, but I have found these to be a bit inaccurate. Even with these tests, it is difficult to pinpoint the exact foods that are bothering people. Sometimes the test gives the impression that a person is intolerant to more foods than they truly are.

As of this date, there is no perfect test or way to determine what foods you are intolerant to and what foods your body likes. The best advice is to pick a plan of action that works for you and start eliminating potentially inflammatory foods. An integrative nutritionist can be invaluable in this process if you need specific guidance.

Journal Time

Take a moment now and write down an action plan for eliminating inflammatory foods from your meal plan. Write down ways that allow you to easily eliminate them. Think of substitute foods and write them down for your shopping list. Create a plan for overcoming cravings for the foods you wish to eliminate. Think of the times that put you "in front" of these foods and ways that you can prevent yourself from eating them, and then write it down.

It is okay if this takes you some time to figure out and fine-tune. The important thing is to start with an action step no matter how small it seems. Keep moving forward toward your goal of optimal health.

EAT THE RIGHT FOODS FOR YOUR BODY

We all need protein, healthy fats, fiber, carbohydrates, vitamins, minerals, and water.

How much you need depends on your body's metabolism and needs, along with your lifestyle.

No matter what you need, what you eat does matter. You may not think it matters today, but it will add up and affect you over time.

I used to say jokingly that I exercised on a regular basis so that I could eat what I wanted. I now humbly know that is not the case. And it never was. Our health status is never about the weight on the scale. It is about body composition and how we feel and function.

Remember, how you do *one* thing is how you do *everything*. You are either moving toward a better you or away from it. By eating the right foods for your body, you are moving toward becoming an optimal you. When you eat the right foods for you, you think better, move better, look better, and feel better.

It took me some time, but I now eat for a purpose, eating the foods that give me the nutrition I need and don't lead to inflammation. I've found that most people live to eat. I eat to live. I follow a meal plan that allows me to build and maintain muscle, to keep my fat content percentage at a healthy level, and more importantly, to feel and look my best.

Always remember that this journey is about making progress, not being perfect. If you can make more rapid changes than I did, kudos to you! If it takes you some time, like it did for me, that is totally fine. Once you are in momentum toward an optimal you, it will become easier to make the changes you need to make. You will want to feel even better and have more of an optimal lifestyle. Let go of the dieter's mindset and adopt a lifestyle mindset for wellness. Build habits that will benefit you for a lifetime.

I remember being in the hospital and my doctor standing in front of me, pleading with me to eat better and to eat foods that were healthier for my body to heal. Even though I had been so sick, I still battled with her because I couldn't see *how* to do it. I didn't know what to do. I believed I had a limited selection of foods I liked and couldn't see the direct connection between the food that I had been eating and the medical predicament that I was in. While I am still "picky" today, I have been able to find foods that I like to eat that are also good for my mind and body. You have the power within you to do the same thing.

I was able to make progress, in part, because of my support system. No matter how smart you are, it helps to have people around you to guide and support you. You can have many people within your support system—family members, an integrative physician, a life coach, a personal trainer, an integrative nutritionist, a hypnotherapist, and more. If you don't have a support system, start with a life or health coach who can help you move in the right direction.

For now, take a moment to go back to your journal and read where you want your health to be a year from now.

Journal
Time

Imagine being the person you desire to be.

Would you be eating the foods you are now if you were that person?

Own the fact that the foods you are eating now are giving you the person you are looking at in the mirror today. Is that person looking, feeling, and functioning at an optimal level?

If the answer is no, then recognize that you must change the foods you eat to achieve the health you desire. If you don't, you cannot move toward becoming an optimal you.

Write down the foods you should be eating. Make sure you write down foods you will actually eat. Start eating more of these foods and less of the unhealthy foods. Ensure you are getting adequate protein, healthy fats, fiber, and healthy carbohydrates within the food you eat. Focus on eating whole foods (foods from nature that are not packaged).

If you can fully comprehend that what you eat greatly impacts how you look and feel, then you are ahead of the game. Most people underestimate the impact food has on their health. Every time you eat think to yourself, *Am I eating this for nutrition, for fun, or for some other reason?* Be honest with yourself. Strive to eat for nutrition at least 80 percent of the time. If you do this, you will make great strides in your nutritional status.

If you are not sure what your body nutritionally requires, this would be a good time to seek the guidance of an integrative nutritionist, a health coach, and/or a physical trainer who understands proper nutrition.

PAY ATTENTION TO WHAT YOU DRINK

Water is the only necessary liquid that you need for optimal wellness.

A good rule of thumb is to drink about half your body weight in ounces of water per day.

For example, if you are 140 pounds, your daily water intake goal would be about seventy ounces. This is a rough guide to ensure that you drink enough water.

Alcohol is a drink that is not necessary. If you enjoy alcohol and want to drink some, limit it to one drink (if you're a woman) or two drinks (if you're a man) in one sitting. Make your goal not to drink on a regular basis. If you find that you cannot live without alcohol, it is time to look at yourself in the mirror and figure out the underlying cause. Seek help from a professional if you feel you cannot control your alcohol intake or if you feel dependent upon it. There is no shame in needing help to create better habits. In fact, it is courageous to get the help that you need to make the necessary changes.

Sodas don't lead to an optimal you either. Stop drinking them. And no, diet sodas aren't the answer. They are full of artificial sweeteners and other chemicals, which we will talk about later in the toxin chapter. If you can't just stop drinking soda, decrease or change to a healthier alternative such as flavored carbonated water or iced tea. Make your goal to eventually stop drinking soda; even if you can't picture doing it at this time, picture it in your future.

I like to call energy drinks heart attacks in a can. Need I say more? If you need energy drinks, there is a deeper problem that you need to address. Do not rely on energy drinks to give you energy. If you have a lack of energy, it is important to fix the problem causing the lack of energy. When I work with patients, I often find that, once their hormones are balanced, they find the energy that was lacking. We'll talk more about hormones in the next chapter.

Drinking coffee may be a treat for you, or it could be an addiction. If you drink a cup a day because you enjoy it, that's fine. However, you don't want to put artificial additives into your coffee. Many creamers contain nasty chemicals. Instead, use almond milk or other natural products to safely change your coffee to a taste that you enjoy. It's also important to use raw sugar or stevia to sweeten, instead of chemical-laden artificial sweeteners. Now, if you can't function without coffee and you rely on coffee to wake up or to feel good, that's another story. If you are dependent on a drink to survive and function, you must look at the underlying problem. Your dependence can reveal a treatable underlying issue.

NUTRITION IS KEY

What you eat and drink affects how you look and feel. It is crucial that you pay attention and find the foods and drinks that serve you well. In this process, you will discover what makes you feel better long-term and what makes you feel worse. Be persistent and focus on what your body needs. Seek professional nutritional guidance if needed.

CHAPTER SUMMARY

Food can be healing or toxic to your body. Eliminate foods that may be causing inflammation in your body. Reintroduce these foods slowly and gently. Pay attention to how your body looks, feels, and functions with certain foods. Avoid the foods that cause problems for your mind and/or body. Follow the Whole30 meal plan or use Dr. Gundry's yes/no food list to guide you, if needed.

There is no magic pill or diet. Avoid fad diets. Focus on giving your body the nutrients it needs. Eat whole foods, avoid processed man-made foods. Focus on long-term lifestyle changes that serve you. Take a ninety-day challenge to get you into momentum and develop lasting habits. Get professional guidance if needed.

What you drink affects your health. Ensure you drink enough water. Eliminate sodas and energy drinks. Minimize or eliminate coffee and alcohol. Fix any underlying issues that are causing fatigue.

Have a healthy mindset toward nutrition. Eat to live, instead of living to eat.

"Take care of your body. It's the only place you have to live."

—JIM ROHN

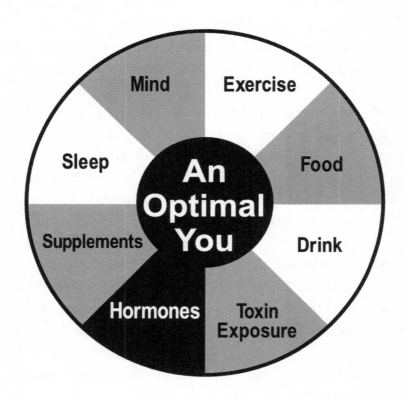

CHAPTER 4

Hormone Balancing for Men and Women

"We age because our hormones decline, our hormones don't decline because we age."

—EMIL TOESCU

"Hormones are very powerful things. We are helpless in their wake."

—MEG CABOT

I received a crash course in how much a hormone imbalance can affect a person's body during my medical journey. A hormone imbalance was a root cause for the fibroids (benign tumors in my uterus). After my hysterectomy, and the final surgery, I ended up in menopause at the age of thirty-eight. I was thrown into a significant hormone imbalance. I remember feeling irritable or moody for no reason. Hot flashes would hit at the oddest times. My sex drive was absolutely gone. It was hard to keep good muscle tone and my zest for life; my mojo had disappeared.

Do you remember getting off a merry-go-round as a child and feeling slightly off-balance? That feeling goes away after a few minutes. But what if it didn't? What if you kept feeling that slightly off feeling? That is what essentially happens internally when your hormones are out of balance.

With a hormone imbalance, both men and women feel "off." They know something is off, but they often do not realize what is causing it. Once they regain their hormone balance it can feel like they found the fountain of youth and can swim in vibrancy and vitality! That is how I felt once my hormones were rebalanced.

One of my patients, who is in her early forties, refers all her friends and family members to our office. For years, she had suffered from insomnia, painful periods, and irritability, along with fatigue and a low metabolism. Once she regained hormone balance, she could not believe the difference. Her mood elevated, her periods normalized, her energy returned, and she was able to build muscle tone and get rid of unwanted fat. She had been told that she was "fine" and that the issues were all in her head. She had no idea how good she could feel once her hormones were rebalanced. This is only one of many stories like that.

Hormone balancing is an important part of the circle of wellness, but how do you know if you have a hormone imbalance?

THE SIGNS OF HORMONE IMBALANCE

Both women and men can know if they have a hormone imbalance using key questions.

WOMEN

- Do you have heavy periods, painful periods, and/or irregular periods?
- Did you have PMS, or do you have it now?
- Did you ever have trouble with infertility?
- Do you get hot flashes or night sweats?
- Do you, or did you ever, have uterine fibroids? Endometriosis? PCOS?
- Did you have postpartum depression?
- Do you have vaginal dryness?

MEN

- Have you had trouble getting morning erections or erections in general?

MEN AND WOMEN

Have you had any of the following:

- A loss of energy?
- Trouble sleeping?
- A loss of muscle tone and/or trouble building muscle?
- Trouble recovering from an exercise workout?
- Difficulty getting a good night's sleep?
- Increased difficulty reducing fat?
- Depression, anxiety, and/or increased irritability? Moodiness?
- A loss of focus and/or decreased memory? Brain fog?
- A loss of libido (sex drive)?
- Decreased motivation?

The list of symptoms of a hormone imbalance goes on and on. This list covers the most common symptoms that I encounter on a regular basis.

For men, the hormonal decline typically starts in their mid-thirties, declining slowly each year without much notice until their late forties or early fifties, when they finally seek help.

I had a forty-two-year-old gentleman come to see me at the prodding of his wife. He complained he had seen less results from the gym even though he exercised regularly and had not changed his meal plan or exercise routine. His motivation and focus had decreased a bit. He felt a little more tired but nothing dramatic. His wife had noticed that he was a bit grumpier lately, but he did not think so. He did notice it was easier to collect belly fat than it had ever been. He still had a strong sex drive and great erections, so he felt his hormone levels were fine. He thought he was just working too hard and not exercising enough.

Luckily, he listened to his wife and got his hormones tested and properly evaluated. Once his hormone levels were optimized and we adjusted a few different things in his circle of wellness, he was amazed at how much better he looked and felt. He saw the muscle tone and strength return, he was happy again, and he had the energy, motivation, and focus to get the things done that he wanted to do. He had his mojo back!

That story is quite typical. Oftentimes, hormone imbalances in men come upon them so gradually that they are missed until much later in life. By catching the imbalance at an earlier point in life, you are saving yourself a lot of grief as you age. Over time, hormone imbalances lead to a slowly deteriorating mind and body. No one wants that!

For women, the hormone imbalance also often starts in the mid-thirties, but women have more dramatic symptoms than men and typically seek help sooner. For men and women, I recommend getting a complete hormone evaluation at the first signs of any changes, or in your mid-thirties.

I am also starting to see more patients in their late teens and twenties present with hormone imbalances. This is likely due to our increasingly toxic environment, which is why toxins and toxin avoidance have their own chapter in this book and their own place in the circle of wellness. No matter your age, if you feel that your hormones are out of balance, get them properly tested and evaluated by a medical provider trained in optimizing hormone levels. Lab costs are typically covered by insurance, or are about $300 to $400 without insurance. The hormone consultation will not be covered by insurance if you are consulting with a physician who is properly trained in bio-identical hormones. A proper hormone evaluation takes time to effectively customize and follow up on a treatment plan, something that insurances simply do not value or pay for. The costs for a hormone consultation will vary based upon the provider you see and where you live. Even though this is an out-of-pocket cost, would you rather have a disease or illness that insurance does pay for or would you rather pay a little bit up front to feel great for as long as possible, preventing certain illnesses and diseases?

WHAT ARE HORMONES?

Many people use the word hormones without truly understanding what hormones are or what they do. Hormones are chemicals made by your body to enable the different parts of your body to communicate with each other.

Imagine that your brain needs to tell a certain cell (cells are the basic building blocks of our bodies) to do something. Have you ever wondered how that's done? Your brain can't just pick up the phone, call the cell, and explain what it wants. Your body uses hormones, or other types of chemical messengers, to transmit the message. These messengers travel through the blood and go to the cell that needs the message, telling the cell what the brain wants it to do. The hormones are like your body's personal postal carriers.

Your body is an amazing machine with many types of hormones. Each hormone carries a unique message, just like each letter you receive in the mail has a different message.

Imagine yourself receiving all kinds of different mail and each piece of mail gives a different direction for you to follow. One letter asks you to get ready for dinner, and you take a specific action to follow that direction. You get another letter that tells you that you need to go to the grocery store, and you proceed to take an entirely different action. Another letter asks you to take out the trash, which causes you to take another action. You are the same person, but you're receiving different messages and therefore respond differently.

This is what happens to your cells. Each cell has the capability of responding in a variety of ways. How the cell responds depends upon the message it receives from the body. The message received is based upon which hormone attaches to the cell. Each hormone is biochemically unique and bonds to a unique receptor in the cell. This is how each hormone delivers a specific message to the cell.

So, how the cells in your body respond depends upon the hormones they receive. This is essentially what hormones do. They carry messages from one part of the body to another, like a sophisticated postal system, sending specific messages so your cells respond appropriately.

You do not need to have a deep understanding of biochemistry to understand the importance of hormone balancing. What is important is to understand that your hormones are chemical messengers that create specific reactions in the cell. When you have a hormone imbalance, it means that you either have too much or too little of a specific hormone. When this happens, your cells get incorrect messages and respond accordingly. This results in the many symptoms listed earlier.

BIO-IDENTICAL HORMONES VS. SYNTHETIC HORMONES

Before we go on, it's important to understand the difference between bio-identical hormones and synthetic hormones. Bio-identical hormones are hormones that are biochemically the same as the hormones that your body makes.

Synthetic hormones, on the other hand, are patented hormones that have a biochemical similarity to the hormones our bodies make but are not exactly the same.

Our bodies are designed to work perfectly with the hormones they make. When we use bio-identical hormones to replace deficient hormones, the message to the cells is identical to what it would be if your body had produced the hormone. This is because the bio-identical hormone messenger, or postal carrier, is an exact duplicate. Therefore, the postal system works as it should.

If we use a synthetic hormone, it is not exactly the same biochemically as the hormone your body makes. To patent a hormone, the manufacturer must make some slight changes to the biochemical structure. You can't patent the natural hormone. This biochemical change can create a big problem. Since your body was not designed to deal with the biochemical structure of the synthetic hormone messenger, the message is not delivered in the same manner.

Since the synthetic hormone is similar to what your body naturally makes, it can produce some of the same responses as the hormone your body naturally produces, but it can also produce some unintended consequences. For example, numerous studies have shown that bio-identical progesterone can be safely used to help control periods in women and help with sleep in both men and women.

There have been some misleading studies about natural progesterone being linked to breast cancer. If you look closely at the data, low natural progesterone is correlated with a higher breast cancer risk. Women who have a higher level of natural progesterone appear to have a lower risk of breast cancer.

The synthetic or chemically altered progesterone, known as progestins, can also help control a woman's periods and is often put into birth control pills. However, progestins (synthetic progesterone) have been strongly linked to an increased risk of breast cancer and other negative side effects. This difference in breast cancer risk is due to the slight biochemical structure difference between the bio-identical and the synthetic progesterone. They do not send the exact same message to the cells in your body.

Sadly, the literature often confuses bio-identical and synthetic hormones and groups them together. This would be like saying men and women are the same. There are obvious differences even though there are some similarities.

Here's the bottom line: the cells in your body know how to recognize and use bio-identical hormones because they are biochemically the same as the hormones that your body makes. The letters (or messages) are identical, and the cells respond the same way.

Doesn't it make sense to use the messaging system that

your body already knows how to use? Of course, and that's why I recommend the use of bio-identical hormones to patients needing hormone balancing. Bio-identical hormones are obtained from compounding pharmacies that customize the hormones you need. I will talk about the different forms of hormones later in this chapter.

Keep in mind that "bio-identical" does not mean the hormones come from humans. It simply means that the hormones are biochemically identical to the hormones your body naturally makes and uses. Under a microscope, you wouldn't be able to tell the difference between the two. A bio-identical hormone is typically made from plant substrates. A plant hormone can be safely and effectively converted into a bio-identical hormone in the laboratory. Your body will accept it, and there will be no unintended consequences.

Some physicians think it doesn't matter whether you use bio-identical or synthetic hormones, that there is no difference in the effect. You now know better. Your cell receptors are extremely sensitive to even the slightest biochemical structural change.

For a moment, let's assume that these people are right, that there is no health difference between the two types of hormones. There still is no harm in taking bio-identical hormones. However, if they're wrong, and it is critically important that the biochemical structure of the hormones that you take are identical to the hormones your body naturally produces, you would be harming your body by taking synthetic hormones.

You be the judge. What makes more sense to you?

I personally believe that bio-identical hormones are the only option. I have seen them work incredibly well within my own body and my patients' bodies. I am not saying that utilizing bio-identical hormones will completely fix all your health challenges. What I am saying is that you should consider utilizing bio-identical hormones prescribed by a well-trained bio-identical hormone specialist if you have the symptoms I listed earlier of a hormone imbalance.

OPTIMAL VS. NORMAL

Oftentimes, I see patients who know that something is "off." They've had their lab work done, and their doctors told them that the lab values are "normal," but they still feel like something isn't right.

I once evaluated a woman who was thirty-six years old. She was having some night sweats and felt depressed, which was not at all like her. She had lost her sex drive and was noticing an increase in fatigue. She was slowly losing muscle tone and noticed her hair and skin feeling dry. She had gained about five to ten pounds that she could not explain. The list goes on.

She got her lab work done and saw her regular doctor. She was told that she was "fine" and that she needed an anti-depressant. Luckily, this woman knew something was off and came in for a hormone consultation. Her labs were not optimal, and she was not "fine." Once her hormones were rebalanced with the use of bio-identical hormones, we adjusted other parts in her circle of wellness. She was able to reduce the extra fat, she was back to her normal happy self, and her hair and skin looked and felt great. She regained her life.

I now have the privilege of hearing these stories often in my office. Many men and women walk around feeling that something is "off" but think their hormones are "fine" because that's what they've been told by their regular doctor. But remember: traditional medical school trains doctors to look at normal values, not at optimal values.

Let's talk about how normal values are obtained. Essentially, the laboratory takes a random group of people that meet the age and sex criteria for what they are testing, and they take blood samples from these people. The laboratory then takes the average of the results and assigns those results as normal values. The people being sampled might be unhealthy but not show outward signs of their lack of health.

Stop and look around you for a moment. Is normal really what you want? I don't want to be at the "normal" standard. That is what I was before I had my surgery, and you remember where it got me!

The normal person these days is overweight, or even obese. Many are sick, tired, depressed, typically on multiple medications, and don't feel great every day.

On the other hand, optimal is beyond "normal." A person in optimal wellness has the energy and vitality to live the life they want. They have good muscle tone, have great focus, are in a good mood, and overall feel great!

Optimal levels may show as "high" when compared to "normal" levels. Do not be alarmed if you are undergoing bio-identical hormone therapy and some of your levels appear elevated. Discuss this with your bio-identical hormone specialist and pay attention to how you feel. Remember that the levels are based on the same laboratory values that often miss a hormone deficiency and are based on "normal" and not "optimal" values.

Would you rather be normal or optimal?

Pay attention to your body and your mind. If you know that something is off, get your laboratory values and symptoms evaluated by a medical practitioner who is trained in bio-identical hormones and integrative medicine.

Any medical professional who is adept at diagnosing and treating hormone imbalances will have spent more than a weekend learning about hormones. Seek out the help of a medical professional who has been adequately trained. I regularly teach other medical professionals to properly diagnose and treat hormone imbalances, so I know that they are out there!

TREATING HORMONE IMBALANCES FOR DIFFERENT HORMONES

There is a wide variety of hormones in your body. When I talk about hormone balancing, I am typically talking about thyroid, estrogen, testosterone, progesterone, cortisol, and growth hormone. These are the hormones that typically get out of balance with our stressful life, poor eating habits, and toxin exposure.

These are the hormones that a bio-identical hormone specialist focuses on rebalancing to give you back your life. There are some other hormones that we may address, but they are minor. My goal is for you to have a basic understanding of the hormones that have the most significant impact. You do not need to know the details of all the hormones, you simply need a basic understanding of these hormones.

Keep in mind: all these hormones can be out of balance in both men and women. There is not a hormone that only men have or only women have.

This list of the effects of the hormones, including side effects and symptoms, is not meant to be comprehensive. I have compiled the most critical information.

PROGESTERONE

Progesterone is important for stimulating healthy bones, skin, and hair. An optimal progesterone level promotes good sleep and helps us stay calm. Progesterone can also act as a diuretic (releases excess water from the body) to relieve swelling.

Signs of a progesterone deficiency can include the following:

Women may have one or more of the following:

- PMS
- Painful and/or heavy periods
- Infertility

Men and women may have:

- Restless legs
- Anxiety
- Nervousness
- Irritability
- Insomnia

Progesterone is often best given at night as it has a sleepy side effect, which is great when someone has insomnia. If you are prone to daytime anxiety, you may benefit from taking progesterone in the morning.

If a woman is still having a menstrual cycle, I typically cycle the progesterone to correlate with the cycle. If men require progesterone, I advise taking it each night—the same frequency as a woman in menopause.

These are general guidelines, and your exact treatment regime must be determined at your consultation.

If you are still groggy in the morning after taking progesterone, the dosage must be adjusted.

ESTROGEN

There is a misconception that estrogen is evil, but that is simply not the case. Both men and women need a certain amount of estrogen to be hormonally balanced and to feel well. Men do have estrogen, but they do not need to replace the estrogen. They just need the estrogen to testosterone ratio to be correct.

Since men do not require estrogen replacement, estrogen replacement therapy is designed for women.

Estrogen has many functions in the body. It regulates the menstrual cycle, supports the growth and regeneration of female reproductive tissues, keeps the pelvic floor strong and healthy, and supports the health of the skin, hair, and bones. Estrogen affects the mood and overall brain function, and it can assist in keeping a healthy libido or sex drive in women.

There is not just one type of estrogen in your body. Estrogen is a group of over thirty related hormones. The three primary estrogen hormones are estradiol, estrone, and estriol. Estradiol is considered the most potent estrogen, and estriol is considered the weakest estrogen. A number of oncologists have promoted the use of estriol in breast cancer patients who require assistance in alleviating the symptoms of menopause. Estrone has been linked to cancer and is not used in hormone replacement therapies. Estriol appears to be protective against cancer and estradiol is believed to be cancer neutral, neither increasing nor decreasing the risk of cancer.

Signs of low estrogen levels:

- Thinning bones, also known as osteopenia or osteoporosis
- Vaginal dryness
- Joint aches
- Low libido
- Hot flashes
- Urine incontinence
- Recurrent urine infections
- Foggy thinking
- Depression
- Anxiety
- Dry, loose, and aging skin

Too much or too little estrogen can affect how you look and feel. Finding the optimal balance is the goal.

Some men need to lower their estrogen because they genetically make too much of it. If a man's hormone system is working optimally, his body will stop making estrogen once his body has the correct amount of estrogen. Some men's bodies do not control the levels adequately, which can result in an excess of estrogen. An excess of estrogen can promote belly fat and moodiness and affect the ability to have an erection. Bio-identical hormone specialists first utilize natural supplements to help keep the estrogen at an optimal level and occasionally need to incorporate a prescription aromatase inhibitor. This is a medication that inhibits the action of the enzyme that creates estrogen from the testosterone. If a man does not have the genetic ability to decrease the action of this enzyme, that is when a prescription aromatase inhibitor is utilized.

I advise all my patients—both men and women—to take the natural supplement DIM. DIM is a plant chemical that naturally helps the hormone balance of testosterone with estrogen in men and women. DIM is found in a pill form, or you can get it from eating broccoli, kale, brussels sprouts, and cabbage. For a lot of people, those foods can bother the intestinal tract, so DIM is typically recommended.

Talk to your medical professional before starting any over-the-counter product.

TESTOSTERONE

Testosterone is typically thought of as a male hormone. Testosterone is also produced by women but in smaller amounts than in men. Testosterone performs a wide variety of functions within the body, and it is critical for both men and women to have enough testosterone.

Testosterone improves mood and memory. I have found testosterone to be one of the best natural antidepressants that exists. It helps increase your muscle tone and allows your body to build muscle and reduce fat. It helps with focus and vitality, increases motivation, improves fatigue, and can even help with improving sleep. For women, testosterone reduces or eliminates night sweats. It assists in building healthy bones and keeping your skin healthy. For men, it can assist with regaining healthy erections.

For men and women, it also has the potential to increase sex drive. Obviously, there are many reasons why someone may have a low sex drive, and a low testosterone level is only one of them. But it can be an important piece to the puzzle.

A man's testosterone level begins a slow but steady decline around age thirty-five. The level decreases by about a percent or two each year. Often men do not notice this decline because they can still have erections and a sex drive. A woman's testosterone also declines in the mid-thirties, but women typically have more dramatic symptoms and seek help earlier than men.

Signs of a testosterone deficiency in men and women:

- Loss of muscle tone
- Decreased focus and concentration
- Lowered motivation
- Decreased memory
- Fatigue
- Irritability, anxiety, moodiness
- Harder time recovering from exercise

- Depression
- Increase in fat and decrease in muscle mass

Men may find that they do not wake up with a morning erection each day and may have trouble with erections in general.

Women may have night sweats.

I typically see men searching for testosterone replacement more often than women, but only after it has decreased to a very low level. Most men do not realize they have a testosterone deficiency until it affects their erections. By reading the list above, you now know the wide variety of symptoms that a testosterone deficiency can cause, and you can seek help before your levels get extremely low.

Women, sadly, are not educated on the importance of this critical hormone for their health so they may not have the testosterone properly balanced if they seek help from a medical professional who is not properly trained in bio-identical hormones. Women need an optimal testosterone level too!

As with anything, it is important to find the right balance with testosterone replacement. Some people search for the magic pill, and they want to take more testosterone than their body needs. This unfortunately gives testosterone a mixed reputation. Remember that hormone balancing is an important piece of your circle of wellness, but it does not fix everything. It is important to address each piece of the circle of wellness thoughtfully and with the guidance of trusted, highly trained professionals.

THYROID

The thyroid is located in the neck, just below the larynx. The thyroid gland takes iodine from the food we eat to convert it into a few different thyroid hormones. The thyroid hormones help control metabolism, regulate temperature and heart rate, allow for fat and carbohydrate metabolism, and keep your hair, skin, and nails healthy.

A low-functioning thyroid gland is extremely common, and women are five times more likely to suffer from low thyroid than men are. When it comes to hormone balancing, we are specifically looking at thyroid deficiency. Too much thyroid hormone, or hyperthyroidism, is a completely different issue and, since it is a diagnosable disease, it needs the help of a different specialist, an endocrinologist.

Signs of a low thyroid hormone level can include:

- Fatigue, especially mid-afternoon fatigue
- Dry skin, dry hair, brittle nails
- Constipation
- Decreased ability to focus

- Hair loss
- Increase in cholesterol
- Unexplained weight gain or an inability to lose weight when doing all the right things

Iodine naturally supports the thyroid, and any iodine deficiency should be corrected. If you require thyroid replacement, you typically want to take it in the morning at least a half hour before you eat or drink anything (except water) or take any supplements. There are several things that can interfere with the absorption of the thyroid medication, such as calcium and iron.

You can get thyroid replacement as T4 or T3. These are two different thyroid hormones that your body makes. T4 is the storage form of thyroid hormone, and T3 is the more active form of thyroid hormone. I typically like to give patients a combination pill that has T4 and T3 in it. However, the specific thyroid medication that you take should be determined by the bio-identical hormone specialist that you are seeing.

Too much thyroid hormone can result in feeling anxious, having palpitations, insomnia, and/or increased headaches. Adjusting the dose rectifies these issues.

CORTISOL

Cortisol is a hormone that is produced from your adrenal

glands. Your adrenal glands are two tiny glands on top of each of your kidneys. The adrenal glands are critical for your health and without them it is difficult to sustain life.

Cortisol is a hormone that gives you energy in times of stress. That is fine during an emergency. But in today's high-stress environment, cortisol can be abnormally elevated for a prolonged period. Our bodies were not designed for that to happen. Prolonged stress can raise your blood pressure and zap your energy over time, among other things. In the short term, high levels of cortisol can also promote weight gain and decrease your immunity.

Cortisol does have some benefits. It increases alertness, energy, mood, and your ability to handle stress. It also reduces inflammation and helps you deal with pain.

However, as I mentioned above, too much cortisol over time can cause abdominal weight gain and chronic fatigue. It can also increase blood sugar levels.

If you are under prolonged stress, and your body produces a high amount of cortisol for a prolonged period, you can get what is called adrenal fatigue. Your adrenal glands, which produce the cortisol, basically get "pooped out." This can affect your adrenal glands' ability to produce different hormones than cortisol, including estrogen and testosterone.

Adrenal fatigue can result in:

- Fatigue
- Insomnia
- Decreased memory
- Increased irritability
- Elevated blood sugar
- Increased belly fat

If this goes on for too long, I have seen some people get to the point where their adrenal glands produce almost no cortisol, and they are severely fatigued to the point that they can no longer work or function at a decent level. In the beginning, when there is an overproduction of cortisol, you may feel on edge, slightly anxious, and yet also feel tired. I call this feeling "wired and tired."

Adrenal fatigue is not typically recognized in traditional medicine, but I have seen too many patients who suffer from it to believe that it is a made-up affliction. Treating adrenal fatigue is not as straightforward as treating the other hormone imbalances. There are entire books focused just on treating adrenal fatigue.

The best way to treat adrenal fatigue is to replace your other deficient hormones that I already mentioned (taking the pressure off your adrenal glands), take B vitamins (sometimes by injection for maximum absorption), take an adrenal support supplement, and implement some significant lifestyle changes. These lifestyle changes include eliminating stressors, meditating daily, avoiding stimulants such as caffeine, eating a healthy whole food diet, and getting adequate sleep.

Restoring your adrenal gland to optimal functioning takes time and patience. Putting yourself first and practicing daily self-care is critical. Your bio-identical hormone specialist can tailor your treatment program for you.

GROWTH HORMONE

Growth hormone has gotten a bad reputation because it has been overused by athletes and bodybuilders who take it at doses much higher than the body requires.

After about the age of thirty, the growth hormone level declines more sharply than other hormones and is even lower in obese individuals. Some people in the anti-aging world feel growth hormone is the magic bullet. There is no magic bullet—you must exercise, eat right, get good sleep, and balance your other hormones before considering growth hormone replacement.

If you truly are low on growth hormone, you may have persistent issues after the above measures are taken.

These symptoms can be:

- Depressed mood
- Decreased memory
- Poor sleep
- Increase in abdominal fat
- Increase in cholesterol
- Overall poor healing
- Increase in aches and pains

Growth hormone controls inflammation and can improve stamina, memory, and the ability to deal with stress. It can improve sleep and it can protect the bones, immunity, and organ systems. Growth hormone helps repair your body from the daily wear and tear of life.

It is my opinion that growth hormone should not be started at the beginning of any hormone balancing regimen. First, work on the multiple areas in the circle of wellness and get your progesterone, estrogen, testosterone, and thyroid optimized. If you continue to have symptoms of low growth hormone, then get the levels tested at that time.

It is possible for growth hormone to stimulate tumor growth in your body, so it is important to take it only if needed and at doses that encourage optimal health. You want it to give you benefits without giving you side effects.

If you have low growth hormone, you may be given the option to take sermorelin along with some other peptides. This is a precursor to growth hormone, and it allows your body to make growth hormone. The benefit of this is that it does not promote tumor growth and it is a lot less expensive than growth hormone. It does take longer to show the same benefits as growth hormone, and some people have found it not to be as potent, or not to work at all. Others prefer this option first due to the increased safety and decreased cost.

If you take growth hormone itself, it is typically about four to five times the cost of the precursors. Both the precursors and growth hormone are given as subcutaneous injections, and they are given in the fat, just under your skin. Typically, the belly area is used, as with insulin injections.

DIFFERENT FORMS OF BIO-IDENTICAL TREATMENTS

I believe in balancing hormones as safely as possible—utilizing bio-identical hormones at the dose that gives you your life back without going too far and causing preventable side effects. Anytime you introduce anything into your body, there is a slight risk of side effects. However, in today's world surrounded by things that disrupt your hormones, it is difficult to feel and look optimal without the use of bio-identical hormone replacement. To minimize any issues, I utilize bio-identical hormones instead of synthetic hormones and use the lowest dose that gives the maximum results.

Each person has a unique makeup of hormones that are specific to their health and bodies. Trust your instincts and know your body. If you feel that your hormones are out of balance, seek the help of a medical professional who is trained in bio-identical hormones. That person will evaluate your symptoms and correlate them with the laboratory values. They will review the hormones that you are deficient in and that need rebalancing and discuss the treatment options with you. You will be given a customized bio-identical therapy regimen.

There are different ways that you can receive bio-identical hormone treatment. Your treatment plan will be designed specifically for you and can be either one form of treatment or a combination of different approaches listed out here.

The hormones are typically obtained through a compounding pharmacy. A compounding pharmacy is a pharmacy that specializes in customizing medication for its clients. They take a bio-identical hormone and can prepare it in the concentration and form that best meets your needs, based upon the recommendations of your bio-identical hormone specialist. Your hormone specialist typically has a relationship with a compounding pharmacy, or a few of them, and can direct you to the appropriate pharmacy. Just like hormones are not created equally, pharmacies differ in their quality.

CREAMS

Creams are a topical application of bio-identical hormones. The hormone is placed within a cream, and the cream is applied to the skin daily. The creams are usually applied either once or twice a day. It is a good idea to try and apply the cream at the same time every day to help you remember to use the creams. The frequency depends on the medication and your needs.

The advantage of a cream is that it is painless, and it is easy to adjust the dosing. The disadvantage is that you must remember to use it on a regular basis and need to be careful about allowing it to absorb before touching another person. You do not want your partner, or your children, to get the cream onto their skin. Typically, the creams absorb within ten to twenty minutes after they are applied. The creams may also take a little longer for you to see optimal results than other methods of hormone administration, but in most patients, optimal levels are eventually achieved.

Hormones that are given as creams are typically progesterone, testosterone, and estrogen. Men typically cannot get enough testosterone in the cream form, unless they are older and/or sedentary.

CAPSULES OR PILLS

These are swallowed as an oral form of the hormones.

Thyroid comes in a pill form, and many regular pharmacies do carry a bio-identical form of thyroid that has both the T3 and T4 thyroid hormone. You do not necessarily need to use a compounding pharmacy. There is no cream, pellet, or injection for thyroid replacement.

The bio-identical hormones that are formulated by compounding pharmacies into capsules are typically progesterone or hydrocortisone. I don't advise taking estrogen or testosterone in oral form. Estrogen taken in an oral form, even bio-identical, must be processed by the liver and can potentially increase your risk of blood clots and liver problems. Testosterone taken orally also can affect the liver negatively. Progesterone and hydrocortisone can be safely taken in an oral form.

PELLETS

Pellets are bio-identical testosterone and/or estradiol that are put into a Tic Tac-sized product. The pellets are made by a compounding pharmacy in a sterile environment; they are tested for purity and to verify the dosage within the pellet.

A pellet insertion is a simple procedure done in the office

of a medical provider trained in pellet insertion. They are inserted into the fatty part right below your hip, in your backside area. The area is numbed with a local anesthetic, and the appropriate number of pellets are inserted into the area. No sutures are necessary. Steri-Strips or a special foam tape is used to close the tiny incision. The procedure is tolerated very well. Men typically need a re-pellet every four to five months and women typically need a re-pellet every three to four months, but each person is different.

With the use of pellets, you do not have to worry about it for the three to five months that it lasts. The pellets absorb directly into the bloodstream and the liver does not need to process them. Pellets give you a sustained level of testosterone and/or estrogen, avoiding the fluctuations that can happen with other treatment methods. Optimal levels of testosterone and estrogen are reached more rapidly with pellets than with creams.

The disadvantages of the pellets are that they come with an increased upfront cost and require a small procedure in the office, and you must avoid exercise for several days afterward: three days for women, seven days for men. You can still walk and carry out normal activities, but avoid things like repeated squatting, running, or weightlifting. Showering after the procedure is fine, but avoid immersing that area in water (a bath, swimming) for the same time that exercise is modified. After the appropriate time (three days for women, seven days for men), there is no activity or water restriction.

For men who need an aromatase inhibitor to keep estrogen levels optimized, the aromatase inhibitor, anastrozole, also comes in pellet form and can be inserted alongside the testosterone pellets. This eliminates the need for you to take an additional pill that accomplishes the same goal if you are a man who requires an aromatase inhibitor. Remember, some men overproduce estrogen, and you want to keep the level of estrogen optimal. Too much estrogen in men can promote belly fat, moodiness, and nipple sensitivity. For those men, I give them pellets that have testosterone and the estrogen blocker. This optimizes the testosterone level while keeping estrogen at a nice low, optimal level.

INJECTIONS

Injections are typically used for testosterone replacement with men. Occasionally women may get a low dose testosterone injection, but most injections have too much testosterone for women and can cause a daily fluctuation in levels, which can promote certain side effects such as acne and mood changes.

The injection site is typically in the gluteal muscles or the upper outer thigh muscle, and you can learn how to do the injection at home, or you can go into a medical office to have it done. The advantage of a testosterone injection is that it is inexpensive, and quickly achieves an optimal level of testosterone in the body. It offers quick results.

The disadvantage of a testosterone injection is that it involves getting a shot on a regular basis and it is not quite bio-identical. Instead, the liver must convert the injected testosterone into a bio-identical form of testosterone. For most healthy men, it is close enough to bio-identical and can be converted quite easily in the liver to bio-identical testosterone, so it is typically not a big issue. Liver enzyme levels do need to be monitored regularly; thus, more frequent lab work is needed.

Injectable testosterone produces more side effects such as acne and mood instability than other forms of testosterone replacement. However, adjusting the frequency and dosage of the testosterone injections usually alleviates these side effects for most men.

OVERVIEW

When you are diagnosed with a hormone imbalance by a medical professional trained in bio-identical hormones, they will review your specific imbalances and give you appropriate options for your treatment. When you see the specialist, they should offer more than one method of hormone administration. You want the hormone treatment tailored to you.

There are some so-called hormone specialists that only give pellets or only prescribe creams. If the only tool in your tool chest is a hammer, everything is a nail. You want customized treatment. Hormone balancing is not a one-size-fits-all treatment. You need to know your options so you can make an informed decision. Before seeing a bio-identical hormone specialist, make sure that their office can offer all these treatment modalities so that you may make the choice that is best for you. Before your consultation you will be asked to get a complete hormone blood panel so that this may be reviewed, along with your symptoms, at your consultation.

Hormones are to our bodies as gas is to our cars. Without gas, your car will not function at all, and with the wrong gas it will function improperly. Without hormones being in balance, your body cannot function optimally. You could have a great engine in your car (or a great meal plan for your body). The oil in your car may be perfect (you take all the right supplements). And, the ignition might be working perfectly (you have a great mindset). But if you do not have the correct gas in the car (your hormones are not in balance), your car (body) will not function optimally.

When it comes to the circle of wellness, many people start

with hormone balancing because it is easy to do. Once you find the right bio-identical hormone specialist, hormone balancing can be the catalyst that allows you to change in many areas. It can bring back the desire and the energy to change what you eat, to increase your exercise, to change your lifestyle, and even to improve your mindset. The lifestyle mentality takes over, and you build habits that give lasting change for your ongoing wellness and vitality.

You may be one of the few lucky ones who does not have a hormone imbalance, but the odds are that you have a hormone imbalance. In today's toxic, stressful world it is difficult to escape this. If you feel something is not quite right, listen to your body.

Take out your journal and write down all the symptoms that you have and compare it to the symptom list I gave you earlier. That can help you see where you might have a hormone imbalance.

Journal
Time

For too many years, I didn't listen. Once I started to heal my mind and body, I realized it was a hormone imbalance that led to the uterine fibroids, which led me to have a complete hysterectomy and thrust me into an early menopause. Ever since then, I've focused on balancing my hormones and maintaining a wonderful hormone balance. As a result, I feel amazing. I regained the energy and motivation I needed to adjust other areas of the circle of wellness.

What I do today on a daily, weekly, and monthly basis to take care of my mind and body is completely different than what I did in my late thirties when my journey began. I didn't make these changes overnight, and neither will you. But the changes are possible and well worth making. Remember, it starts with one step in the right direction. It is all about progress not perfection. Taking positive steps regularly will create patterns of success in your life that will lead to becoming an optimal you. The first step may be getting your hormones tested and properly evaluated by a bio-identical hormone specialist. So, take the step today!

CHAPTER SUMMARY

Bio-identical hormones are not the same as synthetic hormones.

Hormones are your body's chemical messengers.

Optimal hormone blood levels are not the same as normal levels. Normal levels are what most doctors talk about and base their recommendations upon. Optimal levels indicate a blood level people have when they are in optimal wellness. Normal levels indicate a blood level that we see in the general population without any regard to whether people are functioning optimally.

Pay attention to how you feel. If you feel that something is "off," don't ignore it even if you have been told that you are "fine." Write down the symptoms that you have to see if you have a hormone imbalance. Have a complete hormone evaluation by a medical provider trained in bio-identical hormone balancing.

The key hormones in hormone balancing: progesterone, estrogen, testosterone, thyroid, cortisol, and growth hormone. Your treatment regimen is based upon your symptoms and hormone levels—it is customized to you.

Quality matters! Seek the help of a medical professional trained in bio-identical hormones that offers a variety of treatment modalities so that you can have a customized treatment plan.

"To remain oblivious to the hidden regenerative processes inside your body will cause you to die unnecessarily young to our bodies what gas is to our cars. Without a hormone balance, our bodies cannot function properly."

—RAY KURZWEIL AND TERRY GROSSMAN, MD

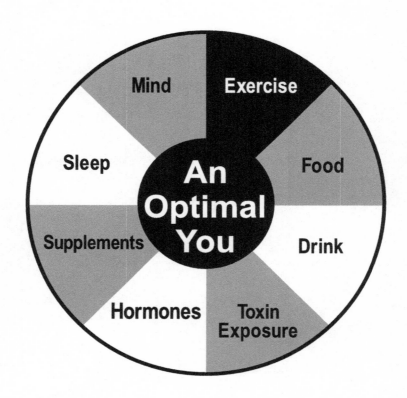

CHAPTER 5

Exercise

BUILD A BODY TO DRIVE YOUR LIFE

"Exercise not only changes your body, it changes your mind, your attitude, and your mood."

—UNKNOWN

"The only place where success comes before work is in the dictionary."

—VIDAL SASSOON

We've all heard that regular exercise is good for us. If you are like most people, you have the best of intentions to exercise but allow life to get in the way. Or you may be among the people who simply choose not to exercise. Or maybe you have a physical ailment that gets in the way or feel that you are too old to start an exercise routine—that the "damage" is done.

It is never too late to start exercising and there are always ways to fit exercise into your schedule, to make it enjoyable, and to work around (and potentially fix) physical ailments.

Regular exercise is an important part of the circle of wellness. Anyone who wants to live well and live long adds exercise into their daily life. It starts with a decision.

The first thing to realize is that any movement is better than no movement. You can start slowly and introduce exercise into your day. It is important for you to understand that exercising on a regular basis is a must if you wish to be an optimal you. Start somewhere and start now! This will create patterns of success that will aid you in changing your lifestyle long-term.

Jim Rohn is one of my favorite personal development gurus. I love his quote that says, "Success is nothing more than a few simple disciplines, practiced every day." Think about that for a moment. How can you embrace this sentiment and use it to motivate you to take small steps on a regular basis?

There was a time during the recovery from my surgery when I could not even lift my cat up, and she only weighed about eight pounds. The thought of even getting up from the couch was a ten-minute decision. It exhausted me to even think about walking from one end of my house to the other. I knew that I had to start moving my body or I would be stuck as a couch potato forever. I had to start somewhere, so I started by simply taking a walk around the house and built up from there. Today, I exercise six days a week and include aerobics, stretching, and weight training. I got there slowly and regained my vitality and my energy over time. It does not matter where you are starting from; what matters is that you start.

You may not be as bad off as I was. You may even be exercising already. Still, it is important to assess where you are today.

So, where are you? You may not be exercising at all, you may be active in the yard, you may be exercising on a regular basis but doing it sporadically, or you may be exercising regularly but only doing one type of exercise. A regular exercise regimen must encompass stretching, aerobics (elevating your heart rate), and weight training (strength training). All three types of exercise will provide different benefits to your mind and body.

Take out your journal and write down what you are currently doing for exercise. Rate it on a scale of one to ten. Be honest with yourself.

Journal
Time

Now, decide and commit to becoming an optimal you. Write down ways you could improve upon what you are already doing. How can you ensure you are doing all three types of exercise regularly? What can you add in and how can you make it work? Write down any ideas that pop into your head.

Before my surgery, I did aerobics on a regular basis, but I did not engage in a proper stretching program or weight training program. What I did helped my heart and cardiovascular system to be in good shape, which helped me survive my medical ordeal. Since my recovery, I have added regular yoga stretches and weight training. Adding yoga has allowed me to calm my mind, lubricate my joints, and increase my flexibility. Adding weight training has allowed my body to build healthy muscle tone and stronger, healthier bones. It has also allowed my body to overcome several physical ailments I had.

Many people avoid weight training due to a physical ailment, but no matter what your physical ailment is, proper weight training can help your body function at a higher level. Having surgeries took a toll on my body. I had weakened abdominal muscles and I was afraid I might develop a hernia. Through proper weight training I have been able to tone my abdominal muscles and help my lower back in the process.

My husband, John, suffered from significant shoulder and neck pain. I first gave him some Prolozone injections, an injection of ozone and nutrients that allows the body to heal itself. He still had some issues. When he added a comprehensive exercise program, designed by our personal trainer, he was able to build up the appropriate muscles and take the strain off his joints. Even though the MRI showed extensive internal damage, using Prolozone, proper nutrition, and an exercise program utilizing all three types of exercise, he has no more shoulder or neck pain. Instead of having surgery that could have caused permanent damage, he was able to rehabilitate his body naturally. This shows the power of utilizing all three types of exercise.

When you do all three of these exercise types (stretching, aerobics, weight training), you will feel and look amazing for years to come. Commit now to incorporating all three of these types of exercise into your life. Make the decision and then figure out how to do it. Don't think; just decide. Commit to being unstoppable in achieving an optimal you!

WHY EXERCISE?

You might know the answer, but let's really talk about it. Understanding the why will help you get motivated and *stay* motivated to exercise long-term.

Remember the chapter on mindset? Go back to your journal and read what you wrote about the health that you desire a year from now. How would it feel to be in that state of

Journal Time

wellness? What would it look like for you? What will it do for your life? How will you impact those you love? Can you see yourself enjoying things because you are in a more optimal state of health? Take a few moments and really see and feel it. Embrace that image and picture it regularly. This will help motivate you and keep you on track.

How do you think about exercise? What words come to mind when you say the word exercise out loud? Pull out that journal where you wrote about your health goals and write down what you think and say. Be honest and jot down those words. There is no right or wrong. The important thing is to recognize what your thoughts are about exercise. These thoughts can help you, or stop you, from achieving your goals.

If you wrote down thoughts such as: "exercise is fun, something I do on a regular basis no matter what, healing, strengthening, important," that is great! That means you have a positive association with exercise. Keep it up! Your mindset about exercise is helpful and the next step is making it a priority, so it stays in your schedule.

If, instead, you wrote down thoughts such as: "exercise is hard, painful, difficult, time consuming," or "I don't like exercise," that is great information to know! Now you realize that your thoughts about exercise are blocking your ability to exercise. You may consciously know that you want to exercise but these thoughts are subconsciously blocking you. Your first step is to change how you think about exercise. Change the words you say to yourself and to others about exercise. See if you can get your mindset into a more positive place when thinking about exercise. Focus on the benefits of exercise and create ways to make it fun and fit into your days.

Take a few minutes and write down more positive words that you could say to yourself and others about exercise. Start utilizing these words; it really does make a difference. It will help you turn exercising from a should into a must.

When you focus on exercise as something that is helpful and beneficial, and you find things to do that you enjoy, it becomes easier. If you are having a challenge doing this, I encourage you to stop struggling and consult a life coach who can help you reframe your thoughts and get you on the right track. Finding a competent trainer who can guide you on the proper exercises and offer emotional support, plus accountability, is also extremely helpful.

The first step is looking at exercise in the right manner. I don't exercise to lose weight, I exercise to maintain my energy, my bones, and my vitality, and to stay healthy. I exercise so that I will never be in the hospital again.

What's your motivation? The motivation to exercise must

be bigger than something like weight loss. Simply exercising for weight loss is not enough. I have talked to many patients at their initial consultation who stopped exercising because they did not see the weight loss that they desired. They stopped doing something that helped them feel better mentally and gave them other physical benefits short- and long-term; they stopped because their motivation to exercise was coming from the wrong place.

The health benefits of exercise do include helping you control your weight, but that should never be the primary motivation to exercise. Regular exercise improves muscle tone and improves metabolism. It reduces your risk of high blood pressure, heart disease, and diabetes. It will improve your mood and increase your energy. It will keep your memory and focus strong as you age. It will keep your bones strong and prevent fractures and falls as you get older. Regular exercise has even been linked to reducing your risk of certain cancers. It helps your sleep, and it can help your sex life.

The list of benefits of regular exercise goes on and on. Regular exercise has been proven to increase your chance of living well and living longer. Living longer without feeling better is not the goal; living longer and feeling better at the same time is the goal.

I am motivated to live well and die gracefully and not dwindle slowly for years like so many people do. I felt what it was like to be sick and frail, and I refuse to go down that path again. I am focused on living, not on simply not dying. Remember: living is NOT the same as not dying. Part of living a vital, healthy life is having a regular exercise regimen that you follow long-term. If you do not add an exercise regimen you are choosing to live a life focused on not dying and are choosing the slowly dwindling health model that is commonplace today. Choose to live!

If you are having a challenge creating a regular exercise regimen that incorporates all three exercise types, it is time to work on your mindset. Adjust how you look at exercise and what exercise can do for you in the short term and long term. Focus on what exercise can do for the whole body and create the mindset of optimal wellness where exercise is a part of who you are.

You can simply start by walking fifteen minutes a day and work up from there. My husband started there and ended up walking a marathon! You may also want to seek the help of a qualified life coach and a personal trainer to get the proper guidance and support.

THREE TYPES OF EXERCISE

In the following sections, I'll review all three types of exercise and why they are important.

STRETCHING

Adding a regular stretching routine to your exercise regime offers a variety of benefits. Stretching regularly benefits your body in many ways.

Stretching:

- Increases the range of motion of your joints
- Increases your flexibility
- Increases blood flow to your muscles
- Improves your posture
- Helps heal and prevent back pain and other injuries to your body
- Calms the mind

Most women typically incorporate a certain amount of stretching into their exercise regime, and men typically ignore this critical part to optimal wellness. If you do not stretch on a regular basis, you are setting your body up for potential injuries and long-term issues.

There are many ways that you can add stretching into your exercise regime. I personally recommend yoga or tai chi. These are mind-body practices that focus on connecting breathing with body movement and they offer wonderful stretching.

There are many types of yoga and for stretching purposes

you can take a basic, gentle yoga class, also called Hatha yoga, so that you may learn how to properly perform the yoga poses. Once you learn the different poses, you can easily add some poses into a daily regime even if you don't have time for a full class.

Tai chi combines slow body movements with balance. It is best to go to a class with a certified instructor so that you can properly learn the poses. Like yoga, you can learn some key tai chi poses that you can incorporate into even the busiest schedule. I do encourage you to participate in a Hatha yoga or tai chi class on a regular basis as well as incorporate some of the poses into your exercise routine once you are competent with the poses.

If you have a physical ailment, you may want to first seek the guidance of a physical therapist. Physical therapists are trained to evaluate your musculoskeletal system and can offer strengthening and stretching exercises that will alleviate, or at least improve, your physical ailment. I have also found that a well-trained and experienced personal trainer can help you with recovering from physical ailments. It is important that you research the personal trainer that you are working with and that they have a good track record. As with physicians, they are not trained the same. A smart personal trainer understands that lifting heavy weights is not the answer. They understand the mechanics of the body and utilize other methods to build muscle strength and tone.

Whatever form of stretching you choose to do, be sure to do it regularly. Stretching puts blood and oxygen into your muscles and ligaments, helping them heal naturally and stay in optimal condition. Make sure that you stretch after your muscles are warmed up properly (blood is flowing to your muscles), as stretching cold muscles could result in injury. You can make sure blood is flowing to your muscles by doing a light aerobic activity such as walking.

AEROBICS

Aerobic exercise elevates your heart rate. Any activity that increases your heart rate is an aerobic exercise.

Engaging in aerobic exercise:

- Helps your mood
- Assists your body in burning fat and calories
- Increases your lung capacity
- Helps keep your heart (cardiovascular system) working efficiently
- Gets critical oxygen to all areas of your body
- Improves your brain function
- Keeps your blood pressure and blood sugars in optimal ranges
- Reduces your risk of heart disease, diabetes, high blood pressure, and even some cancers

Set a minimum goal of thirty minutes of aerobic exercise five days a week. That is 150 minutes total. You are free to do more, but at least ensure that you get the minimum.

The aerobic heart rate zone is 55 to 80 percent of your maximum heart rate. The maximum heart rate is calculated by taking 220 and subtracting your age. For example, if you are fifty years old, your maximum heart rate would be 220 – 50 = 170. To be in the aerobic heart rate zone you would want your heart rate to be at 55 to 85 percent of 170, which is a heart rate of 94 to 144 beats per minute. You can check your pulse yourself or utilize one of the many heart monitors or fit watches that are available. The more vigorous the activity typically is, the higher your heart rate will be. It is advisable not to exceed 85 percent of your maximum heart rate.

In our office we utilize a test called the Bio-Energy test. It is a sophisticated, yet easy-to-do test that analyzes the health of your mitochondria (powerhouses of your cells) and determines your optimal heart rate for fat burning, among other important calculations. You may want to see if a medical provider around you offers this test.

You can reach the aerobic heart rate zone by fast-paced walking, taking an aerobics class, swimming, skiing, cycling, Pilates, dancing, and more. Pick something that is fun for you and that you enjoy doing. Some people can do weight training in a way that also gives them an aerobic exercise. Whatever you pick, commit to doing it for five days a week for thirty minutes. If you can't start at that amount, start with what you can do easily and increase your frequency of exercise over time. Start somewhere; something is better than nothing.

Journal
Time

Make exercising fun by listening to music, a podcast, or a book while you do it. Get a friend to join the exercise with you. Think of ways to make exercising fun and write down everything you can think of in your journal. Look at that list when you need motivation.

WEIGHT TRAINING

This type of exercise utilizes a variety of strength training exercises that develop your muscle tone and strength. Both men and women need weight training.

Weight training uses the force of gravity or the force of physical weights to generate an opposing force for your muscles.

Weight training:

- Improves your posture and keeps your body in balance
- Helps tone, lift, firm, and shape your body by improving muscle tone

- Strengthens your bones
- Increases your overall metabolism, which can lead to a decrease in unwanted fat stores
- Helps you age without becoming frail, you will age and feel great!

Keep in mind that you do not need to lift heavy weights to get the benefits of weight training. In fact, I discourage lifting excessively heavy weights as it can lead to short-term and long-term injuries to your body. You can get the wonderful benefits of weight training without lifting heavy weights.

Weight training can include exercises such as the plank, squats, dips, and push-ups. These use the force of gravity and your body weight to provide the resistance for the weight training. You can add a weight training routine even if you do not have access to a gym or gym equipment. There are no excuses.

If you have access to a gym or gym equipment, you can use free weights and/or you can use machines. Make sure that you are adequately trained on the use of any free weights or machines. I find the use of an experienced, professional personal trainer can be invaluable for helping you develop a quality weight training program. My personal trainer has helped me overcome my fear of using weights, and I now love my weight training routines.

GETTING STARTED

You may be wondering where to go from here. The answer is to start with something that is better than what you are currently doing. If you are currently not exercising at all or rarely exercising, then start with five minutes of exercise a day. Be consistent with this daily, it is only five minutes. You can do sit-ups, push-ups, jumping jacks, and planks. You don't even need to buy special equipment. You can use the chairs in your house. Add some simple stretches once you are warmed up. Start with that and increase as you go.

Next, start incorporating exercise into the activities of your life. Take the stairs instead of the elevator. Park farther away from where you are headed. Do squats or walk around the house or office while you are on hold. Do desk push-ups and dips during breaks at work. Start adding more activity into your life.

If you are exercising regularly, just not enough, then simply commit to add more. Take out your calendar and block out time for you to add exercise to your week. If you currently exercise three days a week, increase it to four days a week. Once that is easy, increase it to five days a week. Ensure that you are doing all three types of exercise: stretching, aerobics, and weight training.

When scheduling your time for the week, think of a jar that you fill with two things—rocks and sand. The rocks represent what you must do. These are the things in your life that are nonnegotiable, meaning that you do what it takes to make sure you get them done. There is no negotiating out of these things. These are typically things like going to work and buying food so that you don't go hungry. If you did not do the things in your life that are the "rocks," you would have significant consequences. Include exercise in this category.

The sand represents things that are optional, that you pour in around the rocks. If you don't do the things that are considered "sand," you don't have significant consequences. Grab your journal and write down the things in your life that are nonnegotiable (the rocks) and write down the things that are optional (the sand).

Journal Time

Making your exercise time nonnegotiable means that nothing interferes with this time. Will you choose to make exercise a rock in your jar? What will it take for you to do that?

Exercise is nonnegotiable in my life. Exercise is a rock in my jar. Exercise is in my mind and on my calendar. No occurrence, other than something that happens to me physically, such as a temporary viral illness, will stop me from exercising. And if something else comes up that I get invited to during my exercise time, I say no or I readjust my exercise time for that day. If someone in my life needs me, I work it around my exercise schedule. When I go on vacation, I continue to exercise. By taking care of myself, I can better take care of the other people in my life. You can also choose to take care of you so that you can live the life that you desire. Prioritize you by making exercise a "rock" in your jar of life.

STAYING ON TRACK SO YOU CAN LIVE LONG AND LIVE WELL

You may want to get an accountability partner or hire a professional, experienced personal trainer. Tell the people you love that you are going to start exercising so they can hold you accountable as well. Make obtainable weekly goals that push you to do more than you are currently doing. It's better to make progress in a slow and steady manner that is sustainable than to burn yourself out doing *everything* right now.

When you move your body with all three types of exercise on a regular basis, you'll see amazing results. Keep track of your progress and reward yourself with something healthy, like a fun trip, a fun outing, or a healthy gift.

What matters is that you do something and stick with it. Start now with what you can and will do. Commit to yourself and start doing it. Then add to it over time, making sure to include stretching, aerobics, and weight training.

If you find yourself overwhelmed, commit to exercising for the next two days and then recommit after those two days are over for another two days, or whatever number of days makes sense to you. This way, you will make goals that you can achieve.

If you find yourself challenged to keep up an exercise regimen, revisit the mindset chapter and consult a life coach who can help you with this. Find an experienced professional trainer who can assist you in staying on track. Exercising is an important part of the wellness circle, and you must do what it takes to incorporate it into your life. You are never too old, and it is never too late to start an exercise program.

CHAPTER SUMMARY

Any movement of your body is better than no movement.

Reframe how you think of exercise. Use different, empowering words to describe exercise. Make it positive. Make exercise fun. Pick things that you like to do and will do.

Incorporate all three types of exercise: stretching, aerobics, and weight training.

Focus on "progress over perfection." Start with an exercise regime that you know is doable for you. You can add to it over time. Start somewhere. Start now. If not now, when?

Seek help if needed! Seek the help of a life coach if you are having a mindset or motivation challenge. Get the help of a professional, experienced personal trainer to design a quality workout program and to be an accountability partner. Tell your friends and family your exercise goals and what you plan to do. Have accountability.

Make your exercise time nonnegotiable. Have your exercise time be a part of your life, something that you don't eliminate when something else comes up.

"Success is the sum of small efforts—repeated day-in and day-out."

—ROBERT COLLIER

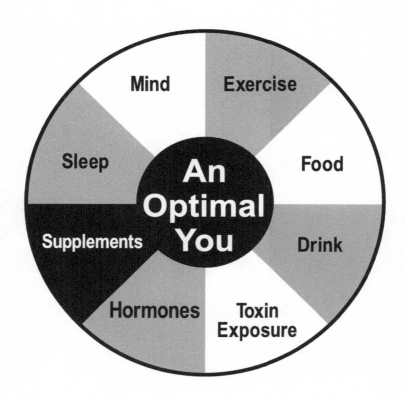

CHAPTER 6

Supplementation to Enhance Your Life

"Supplements are progress enhancers...not progress starters."

—ALWYN COSGROVE

"Nutritional supplements are not a substitute for a nutritionally balanced diet."

—DEEPAK CHOPRA

"Should I take a supplement or not?" That is a common question that I get. I am personally not a fan of taking a bunch of pills, although I do take a few supplements daily. In my search for optimal wellness, I found that I did indeed need some supplements just like the rest of the world does. Adding proper nutritional supplementation to your daily routine is an important part of the wellness circle.

In an ideal world, none of us would need supplements, as we should get all our nutrients from the foods we eat. But we do not live in an ideal world. We live in a world filled with nutrient-poor and calorie-dense processed foods. Our grocery stores are filled with foods that have pesticides and are genetically engineered. Our soil has become deficient of nutrients, and as a result, even the healthy, whole foods have declined in nutritional value. The food we eat today does not have the same nutritional content as the same food eaten a century ago.

In addition, we are continually exposed to toxins: toxins are in what we eat and drink, in the air we breathe, and even in the products we use on our bodies and in our homes. In addition to our nutrient-poor food and toxin exposure, people are more stressed than ever, and that affects our nutrient needs.

The bottom line is that it is a rare person who does not need supplementation. By taking supplements, we can fill the gaps in our nutritional status that are created from the many reasons listed above.

Before I went on my medical journey, I did not give a lot of thought to the supplements I took. I took a general multivitamin that I grabbed from the store and assumed that somebody out there was protecting me and ensuring that the vitamin was providing what the label said it would. I now realize that is not true. All supplements on the shelves are not created equal.

If you want to take supplements that work, make sure that you purchase supplements that meet good manufacturing process (GMP) standards. When a supplement follows the GMP guidelines, it means that the manufacturer has properly evaluated the supplement for purity, quality, strength, and composition of the ingredients. The supplement has been proven safe to take and offers your body what the label says. A quality supplement is one that has been tested by a third-party company to ensure it has the ingredients the label says it has.

In addition, I advise that you buy supplements that have vegan capsules and that are free of gluten, dairy, soy, corn, and any other inflammatory products. Buying supplements that source their ingredients from organic sources minimizes toxin exposure from pesticides.

Through my research, I found a company called Xymogen that sells directly to doctors and that follows the GMP standards and ensures that the supplements they provide are of top quality and provide what the label states. They met all my requirements for a top-quality supplement company. I keep a small variety of supplements in my office that I believe are key for my patients; thus, they do not have to spend hours researching what supplements to buy. I also offer the option to purchase these high-quality supplements directly from the manufacturer through my account. For those who wish to research and find their own supplementation, I advise that you use the guidelines I shared to find the right supplement source.

FIVE KEY SUPPLEMENTS

We are all uniquely different and have different needs; therefore, customized supplementation advice cannot be given without a one-on-one consultation. I encourage you to consult with a qualified health professional for customized guidance. However, there are some supplements that I feel compelled to go over, as I believe that most everyone, if not everyone, needs these supplements. This list is by no means meant to be all-inclusive.

Remember, food comes first. Supplements are there to supplement your meal plan, not to replace it.

SUPPLEMENT ONE: MULTIVITAMIN/MINERAL

Even if you are eating a healthy, well-balanced meal plan, chances are you are missing some critical vitamins and minerals. Since there is no way to exactly know which micronutrients you are deficient in without specialized testing, taking a high-quality multivitamin/mineral is a great place to start. This will help ensure that you are getting the micronutrients that your body needs.

When you buy a multivitamin/mineral from a quality, reputable manufacturer, you will be getting the vitamins and minerals in the proper form that your body can easily absorb. Vitamins and minerals can come in different variations, and it is important to consume the variation that is most easily utilized by your body.

You may have heard of the MTHFR mutation. MTHFR is a gene that allows for the addition of a methyl group to several vitamins and cofactors, including vitamin B6, folate, and vitamin B12, so that they may function properly. If these vitamins are not properly methylated, they can be present in your blood but basically be useless, unable to perform their vital functions in the body. Proper methylation allows your body to detoxify effectively, allowing your body to eliminate toxins and turn them into safer substances that your body can safely remove. It is important to have a properly functioning methylation process within your body.

Therefore, I recommend that your vitamin B6, folate, and vitamin B12 be provided in the methyl form. This way, if you have the MTHFR defect, your body can still utilize the vitamins within your multivitamin. If you are interested in knowing if you have the MTHFR defect, you can have a blood test done to detect this.

A quality multivitamin/mineral should contain a wide

variety of vitamins and minerals, including the B vitamins, vitamin C, iodine, magnesium, calcium, molybdenum, vitamin A, vitamin E, vitamin D, selenium, and zinc. If you are unsure of the multivitamin/mineral to buy, please consult with a trusted professional who is trained in nutritional supplementation.

SUPPLEMENT TWO: VITAMIN D3

Vitamin D is more than a vitamin; it is considered a prohormone because it is converted into a hormone-like substance in your body. Remember: hormones are your body's chemical messengers and are critical for optimal functioning.

People who live in areas with less sunlight or a lot of air pollution can be low in vitamin D. Being obese also contributes to a lower amount of vitamin D; excess fat tissue affects the bioavailability of vitamin D in the body. As we age, our body is less capable of producing enough vitamin D.

Vitamin D is critical for thousands of chemical reactions in your body. Vitamin D enables your body to have a strong immune system; assists in having healthy bones, teeth, and muscles; lowers blood pressure; reduces your risk of diabetes and heart attacks; elevates your mood; increases overall energy; and helps prevent breast, colon, and prostate cancer.

Signs of low vitamin D can be muscle weakness, fatigue,

pain, depression, weak bones, and a poor immune system. In 2020, people with low vitamin D levels had an increased risk of a more severe COVID-19 infection, and people with optimal levels of vitamin D were more likely to have mild infections, if any at all.

Your body can make its own vitamin D when your skin is exposed to sunlight. It requires about fifteen to twenty minutes of sunlight a day. Sunscreen will interfere with that process. Even with adequate sun exposure, most of us are still deficient in vitamin D, and supplementation is required. Vitamin D does not occur naturally in many foods. Food sources high in vitamin D are oily fish, egg yolks, butter, and liver. Most people end up needing to supplement even when eating these foods due to the high demand for vitamin D within their bodies.

Before taking a vitamin D supplement, it is advisable to get a blood test of your vitamin D 25-OH level. Traditional medicine defines a vitamin D 25-OH level in the blood to be normal at about 30 to 70 ng/ml. However, optimal levels of vitamin D 25-OH should be around 60 to 90 ng/ml. These levels provide your body with optimal amounts of vitamin D to perform all its critical functions.

Vitamin D can be replaced as vitamin D2 or vitamin D3. Research has shown that vitamin D2 is less effective than vitamin D3 at increasing your level of vitamin D. It is advisable to purchase vitamin D supplements that come as vitamin D3.

Vitamin D3 is best taken along with vitamin K2, which assists in the absorption and usage of vitamin D. High-quality vitamin D3 supplements will come with vitamin K2. These are both fat-soluble vitamins and they are best taken with a food that has a significant fat content. For this reason, I recommend that you take your vitamin D3/K2 supplement with a meal to enhance absorption.

I routinely advise the addition of 5000 IU (125 mcg) vitamin D3 to my patients. However, it is important that you have your own levels tested and take the proper amount for you.

SUPPLEMENT THREE: PROBIOTIC

Eating the right foods for your body is of course important for your intestinal system. Your intestinal system has its own ecosystem of a mix of bacteria and other microbes. Trillions of bacteria live in your body. These are critical for your health. These bacteria are important for your immune health and proper digestion. Often, the use of antibiotics, eating inflammatory foods, being under chronic stress, and exposure to toxins kills off some of the intestinal bacteria and creates an imbalance inside of our intestines. This can result in gastrointestinal issues (bloating, diarrhea, pain, etc.), immune dysfunction, and infections.

Probiotics are beneficial bacteria, like those normally found in your body. A good probiotic can provide what your intestinal tract needs to regain the proper balance. Choose a probiotic that has at least one billion colony-forming units that contain the genus Bifidobacterium or Saccharomyces boulardii and Lactobacillus. These bacteria have been proven most helpful through research. It is also helpful to take a probiotic that contains a prebiotic, which is food for the bacteria.

The best probiotics are not grown using dairy, yeast, or soy, and do not need to be refrigerated.

I typically recommend that a person take 100 billion units of healthy bacteria a day to heal any intestinal damage or imbalance and take about thirty billion units of healthy bacteria daily to maintain gut health.

You may prefer to consume fermented foods that naturally contain probiotics and help to support the good bacteria in your intestine. Fermented foods are foods like yogurt, kombucha, kefir, sauerkraut, kimchi, tempeh, and miso. However, if you have gastrointestinal issues or immune dysfunction, you most likely require targeted probiotic supplementation that you can't get from food.

These are general recommendations to get you started. Utilize the guidance of your own physician to know the correct amount of probiotic units for you.

SUPPLEMENT FOUR: OMEGA-3 FATTY ACIDS

Omega-3 fatty acids are components of the membrane surrounding each of your cells in your body and are critical for having optimal wellness. Omega-3 fatty acids assist in reducing inflammation in your body, which in turn can reduce the risk of chronic diseases such as cancer, heart disease, and arthritis.

The traditional diet is full of processed foods and not enough foods with omega-3 fatty acids. In fact, most people consume foods that have too much of the omega-6 fatty acids and not enough of the omega-3 fatty acids. This increased ratio of omega-6 to omega-3 fatty acids can be very inflammatory and cause your body to develop chronic diseases.

You can increase the amount of omega-3 fatty acids in your diet by consuming foods high in omega-3 fatty acids. These foods include fish, flaxseed, walnuts, and chia seeds. You can also consume oils, such as flax oil, walnut oil, or Flora Udo's Oil 3-6-9 Blend to get a healthy plant source of omega-3 fatty acids.

Often it is difficult to get adequate omega-3 fatty acids in our diet and a supplement is needed. When you buy an omega-3 supplement, be careful about the exposure to mercury. The fish in our world have sadly been exposed to mercury and any fish or fish products, such as omega-3 fatty acid supplements, can contain mercury. If you buy fish, do some research and buy fish known to be lower in mercury. There is a free site, www.nrdc.org, that offers a convenient wallet card that lists the mercury content in the different fish that is available for purchase or at restaurants so that you can make informed choices. Since omega-3 supplements are sourced from fish, and many of the fish contain mercury, buy supplements that have been tested and certified to be mercury free.

Typically, for general health purposes, about 1000 milligrams of EPA/DHA (omega-3 fatty acids) is sufficient to supplement your diet. For those with multiple sclerosis, rheumatoid arthritis, or any other chronic inflammatory conditions, up to four grams or 4000 milligrams can be effective for reducing inflammation and pain. Please use the guidance of your own personal physician in determining the correct dosage for your needs.

SUPPLEMENT FIVE: MAGNESIUM

Magnesium is an important nutrient that is involved in over 300 biochemical reactions within your body, including metabolizing food, creating fatty acids and proteins, and transmitting nerve impulses. Magnesium deficiency is often overlooked, and the signs of having a deficiency can be subtle. Magnesium plays an important role in energy production and the metabolism of protein, fat, and carbohydrates. It is critical for proper nerve impulse conduction, muscle contraction, and normal heart rhythm. People with magnesium deficiencies may present with fatigue, nausea, numbness and tingling, muscle spasms and cramps, personality changes, dizziness, and even heart arrhythmias.

Having a low magnesium level is extremely common and sadly overlooked in most people. There are several reasons that you may have a low magnesium level. You may be eating a diet that does not provide adequate magnesium. If you do eat enough magnesium, your intestine may not be able to properly absorb magnesium because of stress, poor eating habits, and/or toxin exposure. All three are common in today's world and affect the ability of your intestines to properly absorb nutrients, including magnesium. In addition, if you take any prescription medications, they could potentially interfere with the absorption of magnesium or promote its excretion from the body. All these factors affect your overall magnesium level.

It is believed that most of us have a subclinical deficiency in magnesium. This deficiency can be missed by traditional blood tests because your body can pull magnesium from the bone to replace missing magnesium, thus showing falsely normal magnesium levels in the blood.

Magnesium supplements come in a topical form or as a pill, powder, or liquid. If you are taking an oral version of magnesium, I suggest a chelated version of magnesium because that will ensure that your intestinal tract can properly absorb it and you do not get diarrhea as a side effect.

You may also choose to use a topical magnesium spray or gel, or soak in a tub with magnesium salts, to absorb the magnesium through your skin. The use of topical forms of magnesium has not been as well studied as the use of oral forms of magnesium, but I have seen them provide benefits.

The dose of magnesium needed varies from person to person. Typically, the amount of oral supplementation is 300 to 500 milligrams of magnesium. I have seen people who need higher dosage. Consult your physician or trained nutritional consultant to get the right amount for your needs.

OVERVIEW

Remember that a healthy eating pattern should never be replaced by a supplement. Many people feel that they can eat a poor diet; drink alcohol, sodas, or energy drinks; and even smoke, and they will be fine if they take a supplement.

Nothing could be further from the truth!

Supplementation is not a substitute for eating a healthy, well-balanced meal plan and following a wellness-oriented lifestyle with adequate sleep and exercise. Start with the five key supplements the majority of people need to take, but remember they by no means substitute for a personalized nutritional plan. Taking supplements is a part of the wellness circle, it is not the entire circle.

CHAPTER SUMMARY

Supplements are necessary. The overwhelming majority of people require nutritional supplementation due to the decreased nutritional content of our food, increased stress, and toxin exposure.

Supplements augment a healthy meal plan; they do NOT replace it. Take the supplements you specifically need that meet your requirements to fill in the gaps. Eat a wide variety of healthy foods and utilize supplements to support a healthy meal plan, not as a substitute.

Buy supplements from a quality manufacturer. Research the source of your supplements.

If you wish to order the supplements from the supplier that I use (Xymogen), simply go to Wholescripts.com/register and use the referral code: optimal along with my name as the referring doctor.

The top five supplements that most people need are:

1. Multivitamin/mineral
2. Vitamin D3
3. Probiotic
4. Omega-3 fatty acids
5. Magnesium

"Getting all of the nutrients you need simply cannot be done without supplements."

—DR. STEVEN GUNDRY

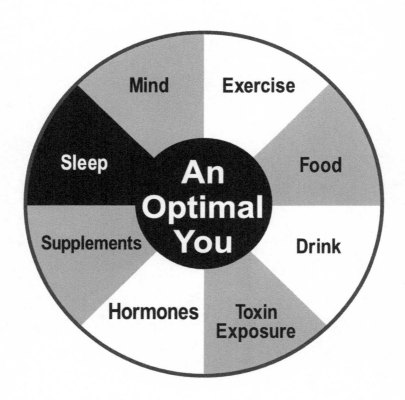

CHAPTER 7

Sleep Well to Have a Great Day

"What good is success if your health has deteriorated from a lack of sleep?"

—ATGW

"A well spent day brings happy sleep."

—LEONARDO DA VINCI

Restful sleep is important. Chronic sleep deprivation is associated with high blood pressure, diabetes, heart disease, obesity, depression, and a decreased sex drive. It has also been associated with an increased chance of accidents and impaired thinking processes, and can cause aged-looking skin. There is no argument that getting regular restful sleep is important for being an optimal you.

Getting a good night's sleep is not an option; it should be a priority for you.

In fact, restful sleep is one of the best gifts you can give yourself. Waking up rested and ready for the day is a great way to start each day.

But what if you are not sleeping well? What if you are waking up tired?

The first step in getting a good night's sleep is to recognize that it is important for your health. It is a critical component of the wellness circle. Oftentimes, people do not get a good night's sleep because they do not make it a priority and they create unhealthy habits that promote poor sleep. No matter what is going on in your life, make sure to allow time to get your sleep. Your short-term and long-term health depend upon it.

The following are other reasons you may not be getting restful sleep and how to address them.

UNDERLYING ISSUES THAT MAY BE AFFECTING YOUR SLEEP

SLEEP APNEA

Sleep apnea is when the airflow to your lungs is obstructed at night. This results in snoring, which is more than just something to annoy your bed partner. Having sleep apnea is like trying to get good sleep while someone is choking you.

If you snore at night or stop breathing for brief periods of time, get a sleep study done. A sleep study can now be done in the comfort of your home and can reliably detect if you are having poor sleep due to nighttime oxygen deprivation.

Mild sleep apnea can often be treated with weight reduction, avoiding alcohol at night, and sleeping on your side. However, if it is significant, then you will need either a BiPAP/CPAP machine or a specialized mouthguard. There is even a surgical procedure if it is medically indicated. Don't fight getting your sleep apnea treated. Swallow your pride and have a proper evaluation and treatment for sleep apnea. Your life is worth it!

RESTLESS LEG SYNDROME

Your legs may move involuntarily while you sleep, which wakes you up at night. You may also notice having this issue during long car rides or plane rides.

Often, optimizing iron levels and magnesium levels can alleviate this issue. Avoiding alcohol and caffeine can help some people with this disorder. There are also medications available for severe cases. Talk to your doctor if you think you have restless leg syndrome.

HORMONAL IMBALANCE

An imbalance of progesterone, testosterone, estrogen, thyroid, and cortisol hormones can affect the quality of your sleep. This can occur in men and women. If you are thirty-five or older and poor sleep is a newer issue for you, have your hormones properly evaluated and balanced by a medical professional trained in bio-identical hormone balancing.

Progesterone specifically is a calming hormone and can assist in helping you fall and stay asleep. Testosterone and estrogen, when balanced, keep your temperature stable at night, which can affect sleep. Keeping cortisol lower at night will help your mind slow down in a manner that promotes sleep. If your cortisol is too high, you will feel anxious and fatigued, or what I call "wired and tired." Too much thyroid can impact the quality of your sleep and too little thyroid can cause daytime fatigue, which then impacts sleep.

Go back to the chapter on hormone balancing if you need a refresher on these hormones. However, if you feel that your hormones are out of balance, there is no substitute for getting your hormones properly evaluated by a hormone specialist. I see patients on a regular basis who suffer from sleep issues and who successfully regain restful sleep once their hormones are properly balanced utilizing bio-identical hormones.

EXCESS CAFFEINE INTAKE

People who don't sleep feel tired, and tired people reach for caffeine and then the caffeine adversely affects the quality of sleep. It's a vicious cycle. Caffeine artificially gives you energy and then later makes you feel more tired. Caffeine stimulates your adrenal glands to overwork, which can lead to a cortisol imbalance, which can affect overall energy and sleep quality. Caffeine can affect your ability to fall asleep and it can cause you to awaken frequently throughout the night.

My advice is to limit yourself to one cup of caffeine in the morning and avoid all caffeine in the afternoon and evening. If you require caffeine to have energy, evaluate the underlying issue of the low energy and resolve that issue. Avoid relying on caffeine to bandage a bigger problem.

ARTIFICIAL LIGHT

Avoid later evening exposure to artificial light—especially TVs and computers. The artificial light from electronics can give our bodies the false signal that it is daytime.

Turn off electronics at least an hour before bedtime. Wear blue-blocking glasses when the sun goes down. These glasses block the blue light while you are watching TV, reading an e-book, or using the computer or phone. The blue light is especially disturbing to your brain's ability to fall asleep appropriately.

PHYSICAL PAIN

Pain can keep you awake. If you have pain in your body, seek help to alleviate the pain.

If it is not something needing surgery, there are many natural and effective treatments for pain: acupuncture, Prolozone, craniosacral treatments, hypnotherapy, CBD, massage, chiropractor, or physical therapy. Get your pain properly evaluated and treated, and you should be sleeping much better.

I have seen numerous patients regain restful sleep after we treated them in my office with Prolozone injections (a safe and effective treatment that stimulates the body to heal itself) and referred them to one or more of the listed modalities to ensure the injury does not recur. Resolve the source of pain and you regain your quality of life along with restful sleep. If you have pain, please have it properly evaluated and treat the underlying cause.

Also, make sure that you have a high-quality mattress that is comfortable to sleep on. We spend more time each day on our mattresses than we do in our cars and yet most people spend very little money and time ensuring that they have a quality mattress. Take the time to research the best mattress for you and invest in a mattress that works well for you.

STRESS

When you feel stressed and worried it can affect your sleep. Regular exercise helps decrease stress. Journaling your concerns can get them off your mind. Working with a life coach can help you with your mindset and give you skills on handling stress. Essential oils can be calming and help you sleep better. Meditation on a regular basis can train your brain to react calmly to stressors.

Set up a schedule of self-care so that you can feel calm despite any life stressor you encounter. Set boundaries with other people and only say yes to the things that you truly want to do. Avoid doing things out of fear, obligation, or guilt. (Go back to the mindset chapter for more on this topic if needed.) Schedule time at a float tank—this is a private tank filled with Epsom salt. Float tanks provide a place to regenerate your body and mind; they take away gravity, sound, and light so that your adrenal glands may reset. Get regular massages or other therapeutic body treatments.

Take your journal out now and write down your self-care plan to prevent yourself from feeling stress. Incorporate this into your life if you have not already done this earlier.

Journal
Time

DIET

Yes, diet affects everything! What you eat not only affects how you look and feel, but it affects your sleep.

Certain foods can impact your ability to sleep soundly. Aged meats, cheeses, nightshade vegetables (potatoes, tomatoes, eggplants, peppers), and refined sugar can all give you a poor night of sleep. Eating a heavy meal before bed can also impact your sleep. If you are confused on the best foods for you, seek the help of an educated nutrition specialist.

INCONSISTENT BEDTIMES

Staying up late and pushing past fatigue is common. It seems like you get more done, but in the long run you are hurting your body and are less productive. When you push yourself to stay up late you may get a burst of energy from a cortisol spike. This will impact your ability to calm down and get to sleep.

You may have been able to get away with this when you were in your twenties but it is not feasible as we get older. Take care of your body by setting a decent bedtime and sticking to it. You will find that you will wake up feeling much better and have a more productive day.

INCONSISTENT WAKE-UP TIMES

It is tempting to sleep in on weekends and on vacations, but waking up at different times can impact your ability to get a proper night's sleep.

If you suffer from insomnia, make sure that you wake up at about the same time each day. This will help train your body to get better sleep at night.

SMOKING

Not only is smoking bad for your health, it is also bad for sleep. Nicotine is a stimulant and can cause you to have a bad night of sleep. It can throw off your circadian clock and greatly reduce the quality of sleep, even if your last smoke was hours before bedtime.

The best thing for your sleep and your overall health is to stop smoking. If you need assistance, hypnotherapy is a proven method with a high success rate. There are also medications that can help.

ALCOHOL

Many people drink alcohol at night thinking it helps them sleep better, but it disrupts the REM sleep. It causes you to wake up frequently through the night. Alcohol can also worsen sleep apnea.

One drink in the evening does not typically affect sleeping. Any more than that and you not only risk adversely affecting your overall health, but you risk a poor night's sleep.

Besides this, many forms of alcohol such as wine, beer, and margaritas provide a calorie-dense source of sugar.

TEMPERATURE

When you sleep, your body aims to achieve a certain internal temperature. It is hard on your body if it is too cold or too hot in the room. Our bodies like it cool at night. The optimal temperature is somewhere between sixty to sixty-eight degrees Fahrenheit, but each person is different. Adjust the temperature in your room until you find the optimal setting.

TIPS TO GET A GREAT NIGHT OF SLEEP

- Go to bed at the same time each night and wake up at the same time each morning. Stick to your bedtime schedule on weekends and vacations.
- Spend an hour before bed relaxing—take a bath, read a book, meditate, etc.
- Avoid caffeine after noon and limit it to one cup in the morning.
- Stop smoking and limit yourself to one alcohol drink in the evening (none is best!).
- Avoid meals two to three hours before bed.
- Avoid using electronic devices for at least an hour before bed.
- Exercise regularly, preferably in the morning and not before bed.
- Limit daytime naps to twenty minutes or less and take them sporadically, not daily.
- Keep your bedroom cool, dark, and quiet (sixty to sixty-eight degrees Fahrenheit is the optimal range for most people).
- Keep a notepad by your bed and release your thoughts if anything comes up during the night.
- Keep a gratitude journal and write in it each morning.
- Avoid watching news and engaging in social media (maximum ten minutes a day if you can't avoid it). And do these things several hours before bed, not right before bed if you can avoid them.

- Listen to a guided meditation or hypnotherapy recording before bed.
- Practice deep breathing exercises—breathing deeply and slowly in and out. If you do wake up, be okay with it and just breathe and relax.
- Avoid turning on your phone for at least an hour after awakening and turn it off a few hours before bed.
- Establish a morning routine that sets your day up for success. Sit quietly and meditate in the morning, even if only for a few minutes. A good night's sleep starts with what you do in the morning. If your mind is more focused in the day, it will be easier to put it to rest at night.

Journal Time

Take out your journal and write down the steps you can start taking now to enhance your sleep quality. Start incorporating them today. You can start with one or two things now and add more over the next few weeks.

You may wonder how much sleep is enough. Each person needs a different amount to function optimally—from six to nine hours with the average being about seven to eight hours. When you can wake up feeling refreshed, without the need for an alarm, then you know that you had a great night's sleep. You should also have the energy to get through your day.

Getting a good night's sleep is an important part of becoming an optimal you. If you follow these tips and still struggle with sleep, please seek professional advice. There are several supplements that can help but they are best recommended on a one-on-one basis. You also want to be evaluated for any underlying issues that could be causing your sleep issues, such as sleep apnea, pain, or a hormone imbalance.

The important thing to do is to recognize the importance of a good night's sleep and make it a priority. Take ownership of your health and adjust your lifestyle to allow for a good night's sleep.

CHAPTER SUMMARY

Getting a good night's sleep is important for your wellness and vitality.

If you are having trouble sleeping, review the list of things that can adversely affect sleep and address the ones that apply to you. Start with the easiest thing to address. Keep addressing things until your sleep quality is improved.

Journal Time

Incorporate the healthy tips on getting a good night's sleep. Take out your journal and write down the things you can start doing to enhance your quality of sleep.

The number of hours required for a good night's sleep varies among people. The right number of hours is the amount that allows you to wake up feeling refreshed. Don't compare yourself to others, focus on how you feel and function.

"Think in the morning. Act in the noon. Eat in the evening. Sleep in the night."

—WILLIAM BLAKE

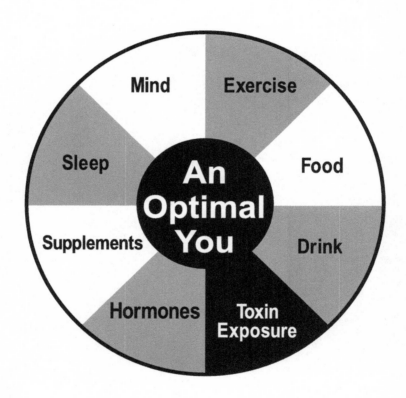

CHAPTER 8

Toxin Avoidance and Detoxification to Heal Your Body

"The elimination of toxins awakens the capacity for renewal."

—DEEPAK CHOPRA

"It's just as important what you put on your skin as what you put in your body."

—PLENI

Once I started regaining my health, I started questioning why hormone imbalances were starting to happen at younger ages in men and women. I did some extensive investigation and found that we are surrounded by toxic elements that affect our hormone balance, along with our overall health status. I discovered that toxin avoidance and detoxification was a critical part of the circle of wellness.

I became extremely interested in the role that toxins play in hormone imbalance when I discovered xenoestrogens (false estrogens). These are chemicals that act like estrogen in the body and can result in estrogen dominance, an elevated level of estrogen. This can occur in men and women.

Xenoestrogens act like estrogen but they are not bio-identical estrogens; they can wreak havoc on your body because they are hormone disruptors. Non-bio-identical hormones can still bind to the cells like the normal hormones, but they are called disruptors because they may stay longer than expected or bind abnormally. When your body is repeatedly exposed to false estrogens, you will eventually suffer from an overload of estrogen. This can create what we call estrogen dominance and can cause an increase in fat storage, moodiness, period irregularities for women, and prostate issues for men. Xenoestrogens are just one type of toxin that we are exposed to on a regular basis.

There are a wide variety of toxins in the food we eat, the water we drink, the products we put on our bodies, and the products we use in our homes. We have organs that help us remove toxins (liver, kidneys, skin, lungs, lymphatic system), but they are overloaded in today's world. Our bodies have not been able to keep up with the significant increase in toxins that surround us.

When I discuss toxins, I am talking about chemicals and

organic compounds that can cause dysfunction within our bodies.

I believe that toxin overload has a lot to do with the increase in the number of cancers, autoimmune diseases, chronic diseases, autism diagnoses, and hormone imbalances as well as the overall decline of health in our society. We have more toxins around us than ever before. We use plastic, herbicides, pesticides, and chemical cleaning products. We use beauty products with toxins that can absorb through our skin. We consume trans fats and artificial colors and sweeteners. People smoke, cars release exhaust, and factories release air pollutants. These and other toxins may be affecting you and you don't even know it.

Toxins can negatively affect your brain, causing poor memory and concentration, irritability, word confusion, moodiness, headaches, and food cravings. Toxin accumulation can make it difficult to get rid of unwanted fat. Toxins can affect your hormone balance. In fact, they can wreak havoc on your entire body.

Most of us encounter toxins daily. In fact, in 2009 the Environmental Working Group (EWG) did a study and evaluated the umbilical cord blood of ten babies. They found more than 230 industrial pollutants in all ten samples. Each one of the babies had lead, mercury, and PCBs (polychlorinated biphenyls) in their umbilical cords. These babies had not eaten, drank, or used any products. They were exposed from their mother's blood. This shows that we are exposed to toxins from the moment we are conceived. Then, once we are born, it has been estimated that we are exposed to sixty-two toxic chemicals in the average home daily, and that is only looking inside our homes, not at what is outside.

Therefore, I believe it's important to educate others on toxin exposure. We cannot obtain optimal wellness without addressing toxin exposure and knowing how to minimize it.

Toxins can potentially:

- Disrupt our hormones
- Cause birth defects
- Affect the function of our nervous system (possibly causing autism and Parkinson's disease)
- Cause certain cancers
- Cause weak bones and muscles
- Cause allergic reactions—asthma, rashes, etc.
- Cause fatigue
- Result in chemical sensitivities
- Cause aches and pains
- Cause eczema, acne, puffy eyes
- Inhibit the ability to reduce excess fat stores

There is a wide range of symptoms that toxin overload can

potentially cause in your body. It is often difficult to determine the exact cause of your symptoms. The smart thing to do is to eliminate toxins as much as possible and improve your body's ability to detoxify.

Each person's body handles toxins differently. This is why some people can seem to smoke, drink, and eat horrible foods and not get cancer or other chronic diseases. The amount of toxins that each person can handle and eliminate from their body is based upon their genetics along with their lifestyle, and how many toxins they are introducing into their body each day.

Imagine you are born with a certain-sized bucket. This bucket holds the toxins that you are exposed to, and if the amount of toxins does not overflow the bucket, your body can safely eliminate the toxins without health problems. You may be born with an eight-ounce bucket, a gallon bucket, or a five-gallon bucket. You have no way of knowing the size of the bucket you are born with. But everyone has a bucket, a capability to deal with a certain amount of toxins.

The first goal is to minimize the amount of toxins that you put into your bucket, and the second goal is to have a detoxification routine that maximizes your body's capability to efficiently eliminate the toxins you cannot avoid. Since you do not know the size of your bucket, it is important to do what you can to keep your toxin load low.

WHERE DO TOXINS COME FROM?

This is a list of some of the most common sources of toxins:

- BPA (bisphenol A is found in plastics, cash register receipt coatings, drink containers, etc.)
- Mercury (often contained in fish, and in old dental fillings)
- PCBs (polychlorinated biphenyls) in paints, plastics, and rubber products
- Artificial food preservatives (MSG, nitrates and nitrites found in processed meats, bromates)
- Artificial food dyes
- Artificial sweeteners (aspartame, sucralose, saccharin, high fructose corn syrup)
- Pesticides (many are powerful neurotoxins)
- Herbicides (glyphosate is especially harmful)
- Fruit sprayed with diphenylamine to prevent browning
- Old paint and old pipes leaking lead into our water supplies and soil
- Synthetic fertilizers putting cadmium into our soil
- Car exhaust and factories
- Medications getting into our water supplies
- Cigarette smoke
- Cleaning chemicals
- Beauty products (can have aldehydes, oxybenzone, parabens, phthalates, triclosan, lead, etc.)
- Aluminum (deodorant, cookware)

I could go on and on, but I want to specifically talk about glyphosate. This is a chemical widely used as part of weed-killing products. Glyphosate is heavily concentrated in all animals and fish since their water and food supply is heavily contaminated. You can consume this toxin when eating non-organic produce and processed foods. Foods rich in non-organic corn, soy, and wheat are especially exposed to high levels of glyphosate and other dangerous pesticides. Glyphosate binds to critical minerals, vitamins, and anti-oxidants in the body, making them unavailable for the body to use.

I first encountered the horrible effects of glyphosate when I met a lady who was in her late fifties. She had sprayed for weeds on a regular basis, not using any sort of body or face protection. She presented with some neurological signs that indicated Parkinson's disease, a debilitating neurologic disorder. She underwent a traditional medical workup with a neurologist and was diagnosed with Parkinson's disease.

When we met, we talked about her chemical exposure and the association of glyphosate with her symptoms. She was willing to try a detoxification program because the traditional medical route was not offering her much hope. We did an extensive detoxification program including nutrition, supplementation, infrared sauna use, regular float tank visits, and IV ozone, Myers' cocktail, and glutathione (these are integrative IV therapies). She also stopped using the weed killer and switched to a natural alternative. She switched to using nontoxic products in her home.

Over time, her neurological symptoms reduced dramatically, and she has only minor issues today. It is amazing how dramatically the chemical had affected her nervous system. Stories like hers make me wonder how many disease diagnoses are missed opportunities for uncovering a toxin exposure, a nutritional deficiency, and/or a hormone imbalance.

HOW TO AVOID TOXINS
EAT FOODS THAT ARE FREE OF TOXINS.

Eat fruits and vegetables that are in season and are organic. Always wash your food no matter if it is organic or not. Avoid using Teflon and aluminum cookware. Store your food in glass instead of plastic. Avoid foods that came from animals that were given antibiotics or hormones. Avoid produce grown using glyphosate or other herbicides/pesticides.

Buy animal products from small farmers who take pride in raising their animals in an organic manner, living on a pasture, and who grow their produce in an organic manner. Eliminate processed foods, artificial sweeteners, and sodas. Reduce your sugar intake.

DRINK MORE WATER.

Water helps your kidneys detoxify your body, flushing toxins out of your body. Avoid caffeine and alcohol, which dehydrate your body. Install a whole house water filter to eliminate potential toxins in your water supply. Avoid drinking out of plastic containers.

USE NONTOXIC HOUSEHOLD CLEANERS.

A great resource is EWG.org. I love this site because it rates the different products and shows which products are safer and which are not. I utilize natural products whenever possible.

Essential oils can be the base for some amazing cleaning products. Utilize the help of a clinical aromatherapist to create safe healthy products that work.

Do an internet search on do-it-yourself housecleaning products. It is amazing what you can make with safe products such as baking soda, corn starch, vinegar, and more.

USE AN AIR CLEANER AT WORK AND AT HOME.

Per the EPA, the average home has as many as five times more pollutants indoors than there are outdoors. Having a quality air cleaner is important to ensure you are not breathing in toxins that can adversely affect your health.

Look for an air cleaner that uses a HEPA filter and will work for the square footage that you have. Buy an air cleaner with the highest CADR (clean air delivery rate number). A higher number means that it removes more particles.

USE NONTOXIC BEAUTY CARE PRODUCTS.

EWG.org is a great resource for finding quality toxin-free products. There are also a lot of products that you can either make or have a clinical aromatherapist make for you. A professional and experienced aesthetician can also guide you to nontoxic beauty care products that are effective.

Since working alongside a clinical aromatherapist and an aesthetician who offer these types of products, I have learned that you can use safe healthy products that also give the beauty benefits you desire.

LIMIT YOUR FISH INTAKE TO LOWER-MERCURY-CONTENT FISH.

You can easily research this online. The larger fish like shark, swordfish, tuna, and marlin tend to have the highest level of mercury. Check www.nrdc.com for data on the mercury content within different fish.

AVOID USING TOXIC WEED KILLERS AND PESTICIDES.
Use natural alternatives. Dihydrogen monoxide is easy to make and safe to use. Salt is another effective and safe herbicide. If you use salt, be sure to apply it directly to the leaves of the weeds and not into the soil as it will harm the plants.

THE NEED FOR DETOXIFICATION

The Centers for Disease Control (CDC) has reported that the average person now has at least 212 environmental chemicals in their blood (things like mercury, lead, cadmium, and industrial chemicals). The World Health Organization has studies claiming that we each have over 700 chemicals in our bodies. It does not matter what the exact number is. What matters is that we are aware of the toxin overload that we all have and take measures to detoxify our bodies. That includes limiting our exposure from this point forward and strengthening our natural detoxification system.

We live in a society that is "buyer beware," meaning that we must do our research and support companies that provide healthy, nontoxic products. Where we spend our money will encourage the production of safer, nontoxic products. This will help us and the generations that follow us.

STRENGTHEN YOUR DETOXIFICATION SYSTEM

Your body has an amazing ability to eliminate toxins and heal itself, but we are surrounded by a huge number of toxins regularly. To have optimal wellness, the first step is to minimize your toxin exposure. But since we can't eliminate or control everything that we are exposed to, the second step is to ensure proper detoxification. You must do both: eliminate/reduce toxin exposure and enhance your body's detoxification process.

It is important to strengthen your body's ability to eliminate toxins so that you can keep yourself from succumbing to certain diseases and other ailments. Detoxification will help you to "empty your bucket" and be able to better handle the toxins that you are exposed to. There are several things that you can do to ensure that your body can properly eliminate the toxins that you can't avoid.

HOW TO DETOXIFY YOUR BODY

Take vitamin C (this may be in your multivitamin as discussed in Chapter 6).

Vitamin C is a potent antioxidant and helps your body flush out toxins. Vitamin C has been one of the most well studied supplements and has been shown to aid in the elimination of many toxins, including lead. Increase your intake of vitamin C-rich foods (citrus fruits and tomatoes are some of the best foods for vitamin C). You can also add a vitamin C supplement. Typically, 500 to 1000 mg daily is recommended.

Utilize an infrared sauna on a regular basis.

Infrared saunas promote a deep, healthy, and natural detoxifying sweat. Your skin is your largest detoxifying organ and can eliminate a large quantity of toxins. Infrared saunas have been shown to help heavy metals, such as mercury, mobilize from your body and be eliminated through your skin.

Far infrared saunas are considered more effective at removing toxins through the skin than traditional saunas. With far infrared saunas, 15 to 20 percent of the sweat contains fat soluble toxins, toxic heavy metals, ammonia, and uric acid.

I personally love Sunlighten saunas, as they have a patented SoloCarbon technology that has been proven to raise core body temperature by two to three degrees, allowing toxins to be expelled.

Stimulate your lymphatic system.

Your lymphatic system is your body's "sewer system." It helps carry the "trash" out, including toxins. This system requires breathing and movement to move the fluids and remove waste from the body. Regular exercise and deep breathing assist with this. In addition, adding dry brushing before you jump in the shower can help stimulate your lymphatic system. This only takes about a minute. Soft bounding for ten minutes a day on a trampoline or rebounder also helps stimulate your lymphatic system and is fun and easy to do.

Soak in an Epsom salt bath or in a bath with magnesium flakes.

Epsom salts help unclog your skin and help remove contaminants from the skin. Your skin is continually removing toxins from your body, which is one of the reasons we sweat.

I personally love going to a local float tank on a regular basis. A float tank offers about 800 pounds of Epsom salt in a quiet, dark, relaxing environment for about seventy-five minutes. Floating in a float tank regularly gives you an opportunity to relax your mind, body, and nervous system. When you relax in a float tank, you give your body the opportunity to focus on healing and your mind the opportunity to unplug.

Eat antioxidant-rich foods (dark green leafy vegetables, red berries, blueberries, and walnuts).

Your body has internal toxins. Free radicals are often created as waste products by your body's normal processes.

Antioxidants help your body neutralize these free radicals, which are toxic to your body.

Take your daily multivitamin/mineral along with omega-3 fatty acids.

Vitamins help your body remove toxins and help rebuild your immune system. Taking a multivitamin/mineral also helps replace vitamin and mineral deficiencies that can be created by toxin exposure. Omega-3 fatty acids also help support detoxification and the elimination of toxins.

Exercise regularly.

Exercise helps your lungs flush out toxins through increased breathing and it helps the skin release toxins as it creates a sweat. Exercise also promotes circulation, increasing blood and lymphatic fluid flow throughout your body, which allows toxins to be taken from the cells and removed through the kidneys, liver, skin, and/or lungs. Regular exercise basically helps your organs cleanse themselves effectively.

Ensure that you get a good night's sleep.

When you sleep, your body can repair itself. Part of this repair is flushing out toxins. A good night's sleep ensures that your body can adequately remove toxins, especially from your brain. Several studies show that the body needs sleep to eliminate waste products from the brain. A lack of eliminating this waste can lead to neurodegenerative diseases, such as Alzheimer's.

Breathe deeply and slowly.

As we inhale and exhale, the act of breathing in and out stimulates the lymphatic system. The lymphatic system is important for toxin removal (it is also important for your immune system). Deep breathing also brings in fresh oxygen and exhales out carbon dioxide and other toxins.

Meditation and yoga can be great ways to help you breathe properly. Our lungs are wonderful detox organs, and deep breathing can help you maximize your lungs.

Get a wellness IV periodically.

I love IV ozone, Myers' cocktail, and glutathione. These wellness IVs are a key component at our office.

IV ozone is a safe process that has been used for more than a century. Ozone is O_3 (three oxygen molecules), different than the air we breathe, which is O_2 (two oxygen molecules). The extra oxygen molecule is highly active and is the basis for the effectiveness of ozone therapy. Ozone therapy has been used to help inactivate bacteria, viruses, fungi, yeast, and protozoa, which are all toxic to the body. It also assists the body to function optimally and is used to help the body fight against autoimmune diseases, atherosclerosis, cancer, and more. With IV ozone, an IV is placed in a vein in your arm and about 500 cc of blood is removed into a sterile IV bag. Medical grade ozone is then infused into your blood, and the ozone-infused blood is put back into your body. It takes about twenty to thirty minutes and is well tolerated.

Myers' cocktail is a special blend of vitamin C, magnesium, and several other B vitamins given to you through an IV and takes about fifteen to twenty minutes. This is a wonderful blend of antioxidants and immune boosters that helps your body function optimally and have proper detoxification.

Glutathione is a great addition to either of those two IVs (all three are often given together). Your liver naturally makes glutathione, but it can easily become depleted. Glutathione is your body's most potent antioxidant and can help your body neutralize toxins.

I enjoy getting wellness IVs as a regular, proactive part of my self-care routine. They can also be used if you are starting to feel sick or if you have other issues such as an autoimmune disease, cancer, heart disease, or heavy metal toxicity.

The exact IV that is best for you should be discussed with your wellness provider.

TOXINS ARE AROUND US

Toxins are a part of today's world. We can ignore them and continue to suffer, or we can face this issue straight on. If you wish to be an optimal you, it is important that you recognize the toxins that you are exposed to and minimize what you can. This is not about being neurotic, it is about being calm and smart about it. In addition, take the appropriate measures to ensure that your natural detoxification pathways are working optimally.

Journal
Time

Take out your journal and write down the known toxins you are exposed to. Next to each item, write down healthy substitutes for those items. If you need help with substitutes, go to EWG.org. Next, write down all the things you will start doing to support your detoxification. Create a plan to detoxify and support your detoxification.

Start today by replacing one item in your household that is toxic with a safer and healthier alternative. Start supporting detoxification by breathing deeply on a regular basis and moving your body more. Add other things for detoxification as you can. Do this regularly and before you know it, you will live in a safer, much less toxic environment.

CHAPTER SUMMARY

We are surrounded by toxins: the food we eat, the air we breathe, the products we use.

Toxin overload presents with a wide variety of symptoms.

We all have a unique "bucket" size. Each person has a different tolerance to how many toxins they can be exposed to before having medical issues. Since we don't know our personal "bucket size," it is important that we all take measures to reduce our toxin exposure and have a detoxification regime.

Write down things you can do to reduce your exposure to toxins and to support your body's detoxification. Refer to the tips to reduce your exposure to toxins and the tips to maximize the detoxification pathways in your body. Start with one thing you can do today and add to what you do on a regular basis.

Utilize EWG.org. This is a great resource for safe products and education on toxins.

"In minds crammed with thoughts, organs clogged with toxins, and bodies stiffened with neglect, there is just no space for anything else."

—ALISON ROSE LEVY

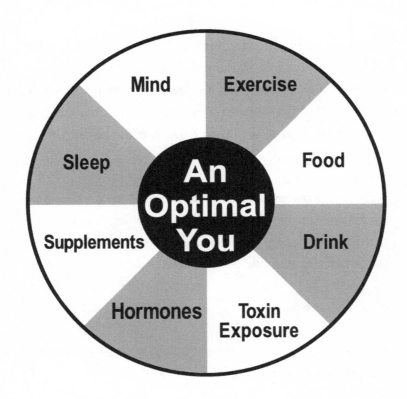

CHAPTER 9

Become an Optimal You to Live Long and Live Well

"The definition of insanity is doing the same thing over and over again and expecting different results."

—UNKNOWN

"Most people have no idea how good their body is designed to feel."

—KEVIN TRUDEAU

You made it! You now see how the full circle of wellness works together. To recap, the components of the circle of wellness are:

- Mindset
- Nutrition
- Hormone balancing
- Exercise
- Supplementation
- Sleep
- Toxin avoidance and detoxification

Each component matters, and what you do with each one affects everything else. What you eat and drink affects your hormones, mindset, ability to exercise, quality of sleep, and toxin exposure. A hormone imbalance affects your ability to get a good night's sleep, your ability and motivation to eat right and exercise, and your mood and overall mindset.

Everything we do within the circle of wellness is connected to everything else. It can serve you, or it can work against you. It all depends upon the actions that you take. Are they toward optimal wellness or are they away from it?

The more you embrace this journey to optimal wellness, the more you can control how you feel daily. You have the power to change the health path you are on, no matter your age or health status. I have seen people in their early eighties regain muscle, vitality, and a joyful attitude.

NOW IS THE TIME TO START

Progress starts with one positive step.

By simply starting a daily routine of taking some quiet time for yourself in the morning and writing in a gratitude journal upon awakening, you can decrease your cortisol levels and change how you approach what you do that day—including what you eat, the choice to exercise, the way you think, and even how you sleep. One simple positive daily habit can make a huge impact on your daily life. One action will soon snowball into even more positive daily habits. Rather than let yourself get overwhelmed with where you are compared to where you want to be, realize that slow and steady wins the race of life. Focus on progress, not perfection.

As I recovered from my surgeries and slowly regained my health, I realized that this information is not common knowledge. Now that you have the knowledge, my question to you is, what are you going to do with it? Are you going to continue to go down the path of slowly deteriorating health and be "surprised" when you have a diagnosis of heart disease, autoimmune disease, or even cancer? Or are you going to take 100 percent ownership of your thoughts and actions and choose the path to an optimal you?

Fourteen years ago I faced death, and at that point I realized the medical profession was content with medicating the population and keeping them from not dying. I faced the fact that traditional medicine was focused on diagnosing and treating diseases, not in figuring out what caused them and rebalancing the body and mind.

You must proactively move out of this system to live. Living means you have the wellness and vitality to enjoy life. Not dying means you're able to breathe and have a heartbeat. I chose to live! What do you choose?

Part of achieving optimal wellness comes through trial and error, and some comes through learning. Over the years, I attended many wellness-based medical conferences. I read book after book and sought out experts who could guide me. I weeded through the information to determine what was helpful. I wrote this book to fast-track your learning and optimal wellness journey.

RETURN TO THE CIRCLE OF WELLNESS

Now that you understand the importance of each component in the circle of wellness, you have a map to help guide you.

The further along I got on my wellness path, I realized that most chronic diseases physicians diagnose could be prevented, and treated, by addressing one or more components within the circle of wellness. The true cause of chronic illnesses such as autoimmune diseases, type 2 diabetes, heart disease, Parkinson's disease, and even cancer can often be directly linked to a component in the circle of wellness.

It is important to remember the circle of wellness from this point on and to keep improving the different parts within the circle so that you can live a long and healthy life. When something feels "off," go back to your circle of wellness, and evaluate what part needs to be worked on. Perhaps you added a food that isn't working for your body, or perhaps you stopped exercising as much, or perhaps you are watching news again and feeling stressed. Whenever something does not feel right within your body, go back to the circle of wellness, and evaluate where you could adjust and improve.

BECOMING AN OPTIMAL YOU

It has been said that life is not measured by the number of breaths that we take, but rather by the moments that take our breath away. Are you willing to make some changes that lead you to a life that gives you more health and vitality, leading to more wondrous moments? Do you want to be an optimal you?

Think of some steps you can start taking now that will get you started in the right direction. If you feel overwhelmed, then start with one or more of these:

- Start meditating in the morning for a few minutes.
- Add jumping jacks for a few minutes after you wake up.
- Take stairs instead of an elevator.
- Add stretching each day—you can do it when on hold or even in the car.
- Park your car farther away from the entrance to where you are going.
- Start writing three things that you are grateful for each morning.
- Look around and appreciate the things that are around you.
- Replace soda with unsweetened iced tea or water.
- Ensure that you drink enough water.
- Use glass instead of plastic.
- Take one product that you use in your house and switch it to something nontoxic.
- Eat a side of vegetables instead of fries or chips.
- Turn off your phone at least an hour before bed and wait a while before turning it on after you wake up.
- Ensure that your bedroom is dark and cool, conducive to good sleep.
- Find a hormone specialist near you and make an appointment to have your hormones tested and properly evaluated.
- Add a multivitamin/mineral each day.

LIVE LONG, LIVE WELL

Take a moment now and review the things that you have written down in your journal as you read this book. Now write down what you will start doing today, or this week.

Journal Time

Write down the things that you know you will do and can do. Put it in your calendar if it will help you stay on track. Then, add to that list over time as those first things will become part of your routine and will no longer be new to you.

These are all easy steps you can take today. Even if you only start with one, it is a start.

Remember: the important thing is to start. If something is still blocking you, now is the time to enlist the help of a support network. If you are unsure where to start, start with a complete hormone balancing evaluation and a life coach to start moving in the right direction. I often see my patients able to make significant changes in all areas of the wellness circle once they get their hormones balanced and their mindset focused on wellness.

If you are already started on your path to optimal wellness and are doing some of these things, then pick some things that take you further down the path of optimal wellness. Keep increasing what you are doing, making it better. Go back to a specific chapter in this book when you have a question, talk to your wellness professional, or get a book that is dedicated to a specific subject to gain more insight about how to keep moving forward.

You have the power to change your health. Take 100 percent responsibility of where your health is today and own the fact that you can control the path that you take. It starts with a decision to change. That is all. The rest will come in the small positive steps you start making as a result of your decision to create lasting change in your life.

Imagine where your health and vitality will be a year from now simply because you made the decision to start down the path to an optimal you today!

Choose NOW to live, rather than settling for not dying. Choose optimal wellness. Choose to be an optimal you!! Be unstoppable! I know that you can achieve anything you decide to focus upon. The power is within you.

Living is embracing life and living in optimal health. Not dying is simply being able to take a breath and having a heartbeat. Choose to truly live, rather than simply exist in the nondying state.

Remember to seek the help of qualified professionals to assist you on your wellness journey. If you live in or near the Riverside County, California, area, or if you need remote assistance due to a lack of resources in your area, you may access our services, and those of our wellness partners, at www.anoptimalyou.com.

"The secret of change is to focus all of your energy not on fighting the old, but on building the new."

—SOCRATES, WAY OF THE PEACEFUL WARRIOR: A
BOOK THAT CHANGES LIVES BY DAN MILLMAN

Resources

HELPFUL WEBSITES

- The website for my office: https://www.anoptimalyou. com. There are a variety of articles and other information about the different areas of the circle of wellness. You may sign up for my free monthly online newsletter by going to the website. *If you are unable to find a bio-identical hormone specialist in your area, we do treat patients remotely who reside anywhere in the USA (as do most of my wellness partners that are also on this website: aromatherapist, hypnotherapist, intuitive consultant, life coach, and more).*
- The website for educational and training courses for patients and practitioners: www.drlaurieblanscet.com. I have created online courses that can be enjoyed from the comfort of your home and at your pace.
- American Academy of Ozone Therapy: https://aaot.us.

This site lists doctors and dentists who have been properly trained in the use of ozone IV therapy as well as Prolozone and other uses of ozone therapy.

- Integrative doctor listings: https://a4m.com and https://acam.org. These sites contain a list of doctors who have been properly trained in bio-identical hormones, and many of them offer wellness IVs. These doctors practice in various parts of the world. Please note that not all of these doctors offer all the forms of bio-identical treatments mentioned in this book. It is important to ask about the specific therapies offered by the office before making an appointment. Avoid offices that only offer one form of treatment as you want your hormone treatment tailored to you.
- Gain functional mobility and end musculoskeletal pain utilizing the Egoscue Method: https://egoscue.com. Egoscue can effectively eliminate chronic pain and assist you in improving your daily function. It can also help you maximize your health and well-being. You can be treated in person or remotely.
- Toxin help: https://www.ewg.org. This is a free site for helping you find safer personal care and cleaning products. The group also helps educate the public on a variety of things including effective water filters, foods that are critical to eat as organic, etc.
- Five-minute journal: https//www.intelligentchange.com. Amazing gratitude journal.
- Happy Jack and his wife offer meditation and yoga

classes online: https://www.happyjackyoga.com. He is one of the most inspiring yoga teachers I have found. He offers monthly and yearly tuition. Great resource if you do not have yoga readily available in your area.

- Infrared sauna: https://www.sunlighten.com. They offer a variety of infrared saunas that have their patented medical grade SoloCarbon heaters.

- Supplements: https://wholescripts.com/register. This site offers Xymogen supplements, a high-quality brand of supplements sold only through doctors' offices. Use the code "Optimal" and Dr. Blanscet as the referring doctor, and you can access the site and directly purchase what you desire. Please utilize the advice of your health professional in determining the correct supplements for you. The publisher and author are not responsible for any specific health or allergy needs that may require medical supervision and are not liable for any liabilities, damages, or negative consequences, real or perceived, from the use of any supplements.

BOOKS FOR MORE IN-DEPTH INFO

ENERGY

Shallenberger, F. *Bursting with Energy*. Basic Health Publications, 2007.

This book reviews the importance of energy and the wellness of our bodies. Dr. Shallenberger designed the bioenergy machine that we use in our office, and this book gives a lot of great information on overall wellness.

HORMONES

Wilson, J. *Adrenal Fatigue*. Smart Publications, 2009.

This book delves into adrenal fatigue and is highly recommended for anyone suffering from day-long fatigue.

Wright, J. & Lenard, L. *Stay Young & Sexy with Bio-Identical Hormone Replacement*. Smart Publications, 2010.

This book gives more in-depth information on bio-identical hormones in an easy-to-understand manner.

MINDSET AND HABIT-FORMING TIPS

Bernoff, M. *Average Sucks: Why You Don't Get What You Want (And What to Do About It)*. Lioncrest Publishing, 2020.

This book is a great primer on helping you get to a better place in your life and health, no matter where you are at now. It is a fun and easy read. Michael Bernoff also offers amazing online and in-person programs to give you the skills you need to attain the life that you want, including optimal wellness. His Call2ACTION program can be accessed anywhere in the USA via phone. His Core Strength Experience is an in-person experience that is life altering. Learn more at www.Michaelbernoff.com.

Elrod, H. *The Miracle Morning*. Hal Elrod International, Inc., 2017.

This book is a must if you need help establishing a healthy morning routine. It is an easy read. It offers great tips for those who are pressed for time and helps you develop a desire for establishing a morning routine.

Grant, J. *The Unstoppable Mindset for Health: How to Have Abundant Vitality Daily*. Amazon, 2018.

This is a wonderful book that will inspire you to make changes in your life and health. It is a quick and easy read that will assist you in creating an unstoppable mindset toward achieving what you desire. John also offers periodic educational and interactive webinars and has an online course that is easily followed so that you can create a wellness mindset. Please visit www.johngrantcoaching.com.

Hay, L. *You Can Heal Your Life*. Hay House, 2004.

This book helps you better understand the mind-body connection and educates you on the specific diseases and how they relate to our emotions and traumas. A fun and informative book.

Olson, J. *The Slight Edge*. Greenleaf Book Group, 2013.

This small book is a quick read and very powerful in helping you solidify the importance of the daily little things. Everyone should read this book. This is a wonderful book to start with.

Robbins, T. *Awaken the Giant Within*. Simon and Schuster Ltd, 2001.

This book lays out Tony Robbins' methods and teaches you how to accomplish whatever it is you desire. It is fairly long, and it takes a commitment to read but it is well worth the time. There are wonderful exercises throughout the book that will help you develop a wellness mindset, among other things. Tony Robbins and his well-trained crew offer a wide variety of helpful programs—online and in person. His Life Mastery program is focused on wellness. His UPW and Date with Destiny programs are focused on mindset. Learn more at www.tonyrobbins.com.

NUTRITION

Gundry, S. *The Plant Paradox*. Harper Collins, 2017.

This is a book for understanding inflammatory foods more thoroughly, as well as toxins. He also has a free yes/no food list that you can access online. The yes foods are foods considered okay to eat and the no foods are considered not okay to eat. It is a great list to follow and will help fix most medical issues related to food.

Virgin, J.J. *The Virgin Diet*. Harlequin, 2012.

This is a book for understanding an overall healthy diet that is geared toward optimal wellness.

William, A. *Medical Medium Cleanse to Heal*. Hay House, 2020.

This is a book to help guide you if you wish to do a periodic cleanse to detoxify your body. He does a great job explaining cleanses and offers several safe, easy-to-follow cleanses. There are many great, healthy recipes that you can use even if you don't undergo a cleanse.

SUPPLEMENTS

Smith, P. *Vitamins: Hype or Hope?* Healthy Living Books, 2004.

This book is a virtual encyclopedia of the different vitamins and minerals, giving great information on each of them. It is easy to read and to follow.

There are numerous other wonderful books out there. These are a few great ones to start with, but don't stop here. Go out and find other great resources for your journey!

My Karma Circle

I would like to thank the phenomenal people who I am grateful to work with.

Alongside me in my office are several wellness practitioners who work with me to offer wellness services to our patients (www.anoptimalyou.com):

Alissa Nazar, RN (Wellness IV therapy)

Emily Stadick, NP (Bio-identical Hormones, Prolozone, & Integrative Medicine)

Sharon Ackerman, PA-C (Bio-identical Hormones, Prolozone, & Integrative Medicine)

We also have several incredible wellness practitioners whom I consider my wellness partners as they work alongside me in an adjoining office. They have independent practices but we work together on the behalf of many patients. (They keep me well too!) (www.anoptimalyou. com/wellnesspartners):

Becky Kay Priest, Intuitive Consultant

Cindy Farrar, Aesthetician

Dr. Donna Ruiz, Acupuncturist, Homeopathic Specialist, & Integrative Pediatrician

John Grant, Life/Results Coach

Micki Jones, Iridologist

Nancy Holguin, Hypnotherapist

Sandra Scutelnicu, Craniosacral and Massage Therapist

Sharon Mayberry, Clinical Aromatherapist

We also have several wonderful wellness practitioners who work closely with my office in the surrounding community. They each help keep my patients and myself in optimal wellness:

Cindy Kelly, Colon Therapist (www.stayaliveandwell.life)

Glee Pozos, Thermographer (www.thermographyinlandempire.com)

Harvest2U, locally grown organic produce delivered (www.Harvest2U.com)

Kori Kryotherapy, Cryotherapy (www.korikryotherapy.com)

Matt Soper, Float tank (www.thefloatx.com)

Rehab House Call, Customized Physical Therapy and Mental Health Support (www.rehabhousecall.org)

Sam Priest, Personal Trainer and Nutrition Specialist (www.SamuelPriest.com)

True Strength and Conditioning, Boxing and Conditioning (www.strengthandconditioning.com)

I appreciate each one of these remarkable individuals. They share my passion for providing the highest quality wellness services. They understand the importance of being an optimal you!

About the Author

DR. LAURIE BLANSCET is a native Californian who married her high school sweetheart while in college. She lives in Southern California and is the mother of several furry children—all cats. Along with her husband, John, she has rescued over 100 cats through the years and placed them into loving homes. She enjoys traveling, scuba diving, reading, and personal development, but her greatest passion lies in promoting wellness—both for herself and her patients.

Laurie became a board-certified family physician in 1999 and later transitioned to an integrative medical practice in 2012 after barely surviving her own medical journey. This journey led her to wellness, which resulted in the transformation of her health and wellbeing. She feels better now in her '50s than she did in her '30s!

Since her transformation, she has been able to help her patients achieve wellness in a way that wasn't previously possible in traditional, insurance-based medical practices. As horrible as it was at the time, she is eternally thankful for her medical journey because she learned the simple secrets to live long and live well and now can teach them to others.

It is her passion to change how medicine is practiced so that it is focused on assisting people in feeling and looking optimal, something that is beyond what is considered "normal". She believes that everyone can live long AND live well. To connect with Laurie and learn more about the training she offers for all types of health professionals, visit www.drlaurieblanscet.com. She also offers online courses that help you to further your personal wellness journey that she has outlined in this book at www.drlaurieblanscet.com. For patient care appointments, contact her office at www.anoptimalyou.com.